ADVANCED AUTOGENIC TRAINING AND PRIMAL AWARENESS

"James Endredy continues to tap into the primordial ways of healing. *Advanced Autogenic Training and Primal Awareness* is a marriage of his power of storytelling and his vast personal history with the practice. It is not often in this lifetime that one meets a true spiritual master, but this generation has James, and this book is a must-have for those desirous of deepening their connection with the I AM."

SHAWN TASSONE, M.D., PH.D., COAUTHOR OF
SPIRITUAL PREGNANCY: DEVELOP, NURTURE &
EMBRACE THE JOURNEY TO MOTHERHOOD

ADVANCED AUTOGENIC TRAINING AND PRIMAL AWARENESS

TECHNIQUES FOR WELLNESS, DEEPER CONNECTION TO NATURE, AND HIGHER CONSCIOUSNESS

JAMES ENDREDY

Bear & Company

Rochester, Vermont • Toronto, Canada

Bear & Company
One Park Street
Rochester, Vermont 05767
www.BearandCompanyBooks.com

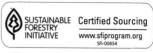

Text stock is SFI certified

Bear & Company is a division of Inner Traditions International

*Note to the reader: This book is intended as an informational guide. The remedies,
approaches, and techniques described herein are meant to supplement, and not to be a
substitute for, professional medical care or treatment. They should not be used to treat a
serious ailment without prior consultation with a qualified health care professional.*

Library of Congress Cataloging-in-Publication Data
Names: Endredy, James, author.
Title: Advanced autogenic training and primal awareness : techniques for
    wellness, deeper connection to nature, and higher consciousness / James Endredy.
Description: Rochester, Vermont : Bear & Company , [2016] | Includes
    bibliographical references and index.
Identifiers: LCCN 2016000326 (print) | LCCN 2016011406 (e-book) |
    ISBN 9781591432456 (paperback) | ISBN 9781591432463 (e-book)
Subjects: LCSH: Autogenic training—Popular works. | Mind and body—Popular
    works. | Self-care, Health—Popular works. | BISAC: BODY, MIND & SPIRIT /
    Gaia & Earth Energies. | SELF-HELP / Spiritual. | HEALTH & FITNESS /
    Alternative Therapies.
Classification: LCC RC499.A8 E53 2016 (print) | LCC RC499.A8 (e-book) | DDC
    615.8/5122—dc23
LC record available at http://lccn.loc.gov/2016000326

Printed and bound in the United States by Lake Book Manufacturing, Inc.
The text stock is SFI certified. The Sustainable Forestry Initiative® program promotes
sustainable forest management.

10 9 8 7 6 5 4 3 2 1

Text design and layout by Virginia Scott Bowman
This book was typeset in Garamond Premire Pro, Gill Sans, and Helvetica Neue with
Trajan Pro and Covington Condensed used as display typefaces

To send correspondence to the author of this book, mail a first-class letter to the author
c/o Inner Traditions • Bear & Company, One Park Street, Rochester, VT 05767, and we
will forward the communication, or contact the author directly at **jamesendredy.com**.

CONTENTS

PART THREE
Advanced Autogenic Training Techniques

PART FOUR
Techniques of Primal Mind, Autogenic Training, Our Senses, and the Natural World

ACKNOWLEDGMENTS

Special thanks to Jacki and Sasha for providing me with the most excellent place and environment for the writing of this book.

To all the participants of my classes and workshops, your continued involvement and contributions have helped take my work to higher levels—thank you!

Once again I extend my appreciation and gratitude to my friends and colleagues at Inner Traditions • Bear & Co. for the continued support of my work and the amazing job you all do.

This book is an extension of my teachers—Johannes Scheuerman, who originally introduced me to and taught me autogenic training, and my primal mind mentors, the elders and shaman of the Huichol/Wirrarika, Seneca, Lenni Lenape, Apurimac Inca, Arapaho, Minnecojou Sioux, Kanaka Maoli, Tuscarora, Tukano, Mazatek, Yurok, Navaho, Hopi, and Yucatec Maya. Many blessings to all these wonderfully grounded healers and teachers.

What Is the Goal of This Book?

I first began learning about autogenic training (AT) and primal mind awareness (PM) before I even knew what they were. Between the ages of about four through thirteen, living in semirural Pennsylvania, I had many experiences with my body, with nature and animals, and especially with my mind, that I can now say fell into both categories. During the course of my adult life I have been blessed with opportunities to live and learn from primal cultures throughout the globe while also studying with shamans, lamas, siddhas, road men, medicine women, and leaders in the modern fields of ecopsychology, naturopathy, autogenic training, biofeedback, bioregionalism, and sustainable living. For those of you not aware of my previous eight books, they all include experiences and practices of both AT and PM, although I did not label them as such.

I believe that autogenic training and primal mind awareness can serve as a catalyst for humanity's evolution. I realize this is a bold statement, but it stems from my own direct experience, derived from over twenty-five years living and learning from primal cultures and then translating those experiences into something valuable for modern Westerners. It is my hope that by sharing this information a seed will be planted that will grow roots and branches both deep and high, so that others can take my work and these ideas to the next level. My intention in providing this material is for others to draw from it, expand on it, go for it, and make it real in their own lives.

In this book I will address the following:

- How AT and PM are defined and the mechanisms that activate them
- Where these techniques come from
- How they overlap or differ from other methods that are seemingly similar in their approaches and objectives
- Who can benefit from these techniques
- How they are learned
- How they can be taught to others
- Forty specific techniques and exercises of both autogenic training and primal mind that are based on my personal experiences and those of my counseling clients and participants in my personal-growth workshops

Do these techniques really work? Do they produce quantifiable transformation? Are the effects of AT and PM long-lasting? Are AT and PM useful for people not addressing a specific psychological or physiological problem? In compiling this book, these are some of the questions I had in mind. To provide answers, I have divided this book into four parts with a total of forty training exercises. The first part addresses the meaning, history, philosophy, and usefulness of autogenic training and primal mind awareness. The second part reveals the experiential techniques of AT, including the standard AT formulas as well as affirmation and healing formulas. Advanced techniques of visualization, meditation, and our energetic tunnels, or chakras, are presented in the third part. The fourth part of the book combines autogenic training and primal mind trainings related to our senses, to the world of nature, and to rites of passage. All four parts of the book include detailed training techniques that provide experiences for optimizing health and self-awareness and expanding consciousness.

This book is intended as a how-to for those interested in (seemingly) esoteric practices that promote higher awareness and optimal health. But far from being a sterile, clinical catalog, this material is presented, I believe, in a way that will hold your interest and at times even amuse you. Honestly, many of the techniques presented here can be thoroughly exhilarating and could even lead to peak experiences.* Other techniques can be excruciatingly boring—that is, until you actually feel their results. The main goal of this book then is to provide you with information—hopefully in a thoroughly engaging way—that can be incorporated into your own life in a practical way. This could mean sticking to the techniques exactly as I have described them, adding them to practices you are already engaged in or, after experiencing deep facets of AT and PM, developing your own techniques.

---

*Abraham Maslow's concise book *Religions, Values, and Peak-Experiences* is one of my all-time favorites in this genre and I highly recommended it. Maslow coined the term *peak experiences,* describing them as "rare, exciting, oceanic, deeply moving, exhilarating, elevating experiences that generate an advanced form of perceiving reality, and are even mystic and magical in their effect upon the experimenter."

PART ONE

Introduction to
Autogenic Training and
Primal Mind Awareness

1

WHAT IS AUTOGENIC TRAINING?

To begin, it is extremely important to clearly understand the definition of the word *autogenic* and its implications. The prefix *auto* means "by yourself"; *genic* means "generated." Therefore, the etymology of *autogenic* implies "produced from within," "self-generating." In this book I'm going to first familiarize you with autogenic training (AT) in its historical, classical sense. I will then introduce you to my transmuted and comprehensive modern version of AT that adds the component of primal mind (PM) to this form of self-generated training.

Autogenic training as it is classically understood is credited to Johannes Heinrich Schultz (1884–1970), a German physician, psychiatrist, and professor who was fascinated with the practice of hypnosis but couldn't initially spend much time on it because hypnotherapy was considered an ersatz professional technique in Schultz's era. The time period between the two world wars was dominated by psychoanalysis, considered the respected and effective mental therapeutic tool. Thus it came to be that Schultz went into private practice to do his work, and some years later, in 1932, he published the first book on autogenic training.

Schultz first developed AT based on his own experiences with clinical hypnosis, which he combined with the brain research of physician and neurologist Oscar Vogt (1870–1959), who at that time had considerable influence on the neurological sciences worldwide. Vogt reportedly explained to Schultz that his patients could produce sensations of heaviness and warmth through mental concentration by "switching" from normal awareness into a self-hypnotic trance, which he termed *autohypnosis*. Vogt's reports and Schultz's own experiences with his hypnotized patients led him to a revolutionary conclusion: hypnosis was not the result of the hypnotist acting on the patient but was instead the result of the patient wanting or permitting it to happen. This was the birth of Schultz's concept of self-generated training, or AT. Throughout the following years, Schultz developed techniques to reliably induce self-regulation and sensations in various parts of the body.

Schultz developed the basics of AT by combining the concept of autohypnosis with specific techniques to integrate mental and physical functions. These techniques induced deep states of mental and physiological relaxation. Schultz's next step was to take people experienced in inducing these deep states of relaxation to the next level, into passive concentration. In 1953 he described AT as a "method of rational physiological exercises designed to produce a general psychobiological reorganization."[1]

Autogenic training is unique because it embraces the new paradox (at least new in Western cultures) of passive concentration, or what is known as *passive volition* (I prefer the latter term). In classical autogenic training, volition—the act of making a choice or decision—is definitely applied, but not the *will of action*. The concept of passive volition is best explained by examples. As you will see shortly in the classical technique of AT, one of the first steps is to feel your hands becoming warmer. However, if you try to force yourself by means of your own will to feel your hands warming, they will not. They will either stay the same or even become cooler. Techniques of classical AT say to simply tell your body what to do, and then get out of your own way and allow your body to do it.

Falling asleep is a good example of passive volition that we all know well. Have you ever tried to force yourself to go to sleep? Did it work?

I'm guessing probably not. The harder we try to fall asleep, the more awake we become. By knowing we want or need to sleep and then simply relaxing, becoming quiet in both mind and body, and even visualizing being asleep, we plant the seed of sleep and allow our psychophysiological organism to do the rest. AT further explores the phenomenon of passive volition by using this technique to affect our normally involuntary and unconscious processes.

In attempting to explain this better I have found the work of some researchers in the field of biofeedback to be helpful. For example, Elmer and Alyce Green, pioneers in the field of biofeedback, have this to say about passive volition: "A metaphoric way of putting it is to say that the cortex plants the idea in the subcortex and then allows nature to take its course without interference."[2] The Greens go on to explain that passive volition can be seen as being analogous to farming. The analogy goes something like this: (a) a farmer desires and visualizes a crop of corn; so (b) he carefully plants his seeds in the earth; then (c) he allows nature to take its course; and finally (d) he obtains the corn. Correspondingly, employing passive volition to affect our normally involuntary or unconscious processes looks like this: (a) we desire a certain mental or physiological behavior (conscious cortical process); so (b) we plant the idea in the psychological earth of our being (the subcortical area); then (c) we let nature take its course without interfering (if the farmer digs up his seeds to check on them they will never grow); and finally (d) we reap an enhanced experience of life.

THE NERVOUS SYSTEM: AN OVERVIEW

So far we have brought to light the original creator of AT, and that classical AT integrates mental and physical functions with self-generated training and accomplishes this through affecting our normally involuntary and unconscious processes through the paradox of passive volition. Our involuntary and unconscious processes pertaining to classical AT happen scientifically in the sympathetic and parasympathetic regions of the autonomic nervous system. For this reason, a short discussion about the nervous system is essential to understanding AT.

The nervous system has two major fields: the central nervous system (CNS) is the command center of the human organism and includes the brain and spinal cord; the peripheral nervous system (PNS) is the part of the nervous system that consists of the nerves and ganglia outside of the brain and spinal cord. Classical AT deals primarily with the PNS. The main function of the PNS is to connect the CNS to the limbs and organs, essentially serving as a communication relay going back and forth between the brain and the extremities. Unlike the CNS, the PNS is not protected by the bones of the spine and skull or by the blood-brain barrier, which leaves it exposed to toxins and mechanical injuries.

The PNS is further divided into the somatic nervous system (SoNS) and the autonomic nervous system (ANS). The SoNS is the part of the peripheral nervous system associated with the voluntary control of body movements via skeletal muscles. The ANS, also known as the *visceral nervous system,* or *involuntary nervous system,* is the part of the peripheral nervous system that acts as a control system that functions largely below the level of consciousness to regulate visceral functions such as heart rate, digestion, respiration, salivation, perspiration, pupillary dilation, micturition (urination), sexual arousal, breathing, and swallowing. Most autonomous functions are involuntary, but they can often work in conjunction with the somatic nervous system, which provides voluntary control. Classical autogenic training focuses techniques toward the ANS, which is further divided into two systems.

Within the brain, the ANS is located in the medulla oblongata in the lower brain stem. The medulla's major ANS functions include respiration (the respiratory control center, or RCC), cardiac regulation (the cardiac control center, or CCC), vasomotor activity (the vasomotor center, or VMC), and certain reflex actions (such as coughing, sneezing, vomiting, and swallowing). Those are then subdivided into other areas and are also linked to ANS subsystems and nervous systems external to the brain. The hypothalamus, just above the brain stem, acts as an integrator for autonomic functions, receiving ANS regulatory input from the limbic system (or paleomammalian brain) to do so. More about the all-important limbic system soon.

So here is the part we are most interested in as concerns AT: The ANS is divided into two main subsystems, the parasympathetic nervous system (PSNS) and the sympathetic nervous system (SNS). Depending on the circumstances, these subsystems may operate independently of each other or interact cooperatively. The SNS is considered the "fight-or-flight" system, while the PSNS is often considered the "rest and digest" or "feed and breed" system. In many cases, PSNS and SNS have opposing actions, wherein one system activates a physiological response and the other inhibits it. The modern characterization is that the sympathetic nervous system is a quick-response mobilizing system, and the parasympathetic is a more slowly activated, dampening system, but even this characterization has exceptions, such as in sexual arousal and orgasm, wherein both play a role.

In general, ANS functions can be divided into sensory (afferent) and motor (efferent) subsystems. Within both, there are inhibitory and excitatory synapses between neurons. Relatively recently, a third subsystem of neurons that have been named *nonadrenergic and noncholinergic neurons* (because they use nitric oxide as a neurotransmitter) have been described and found to be integral in autonomic function, in particular in the gut and the lungs.

Classical autogenic training centers on the self-regulating portions of the autonomic nervous system, which now brings us to a very big point about AT: homeostasis. This describes the property of a system in which variables are regulated so that internal conditions remain stable and relatively constant. Although the term *homeostasis* was originally used to refer to processes within living organisms, it is also frequently applied to automatic control systems like a thermostat, which operates by switching heaters or air conditioners on and off in response to the output of a temperature sensor; the cruise control of a car, which adjusts the car's throttle in response to changes in speed; and an autopilot, which operates the steering controls of an aircraft or ship in response to deviation from a preset compass bearing or route.

This similarly occurs in our ANS as the sympathetic nervous system operates jointly with the parasympathetic nervous system (see figures 1.1 and 1.2) to maintain visceral functioning. But we must keep in mind that if perfect homeostasis could be achieved and sustained physiologically, with nothing else to interfere, there would be no diseases and we would probably not even die. Of course, this is not the reality we live in. What really happens is that the ANS homeostasis is constantly being affected by the CNS control center, which is continuously dealing with the changing demands of life. When the

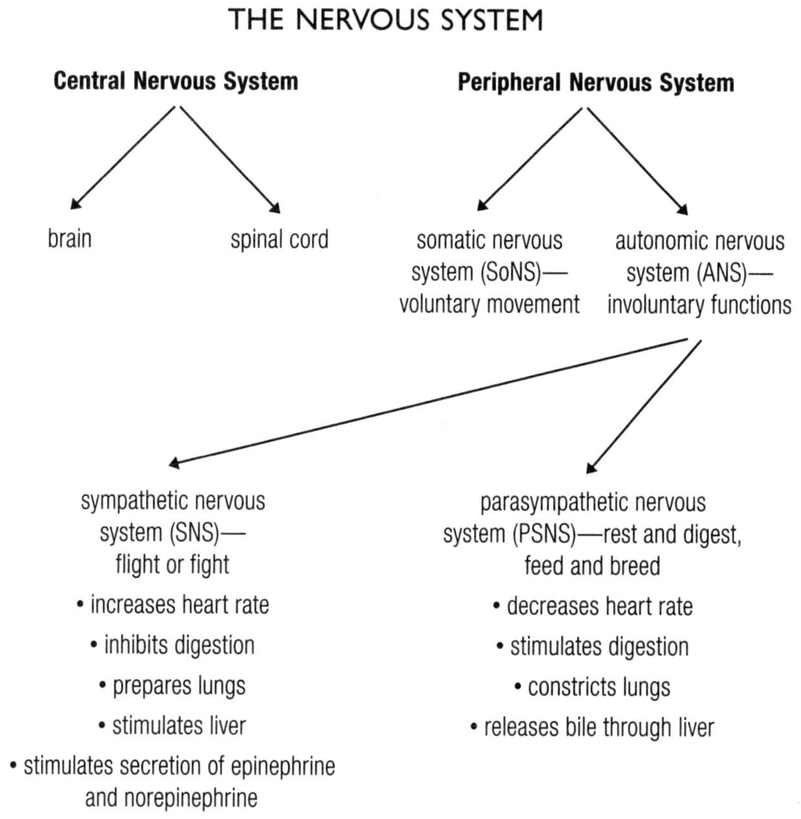

THE NERVOUS SYSTEM

Central Nervous System

brain   spinal cord

Peripheral Nervous System

somatic nervous   autonomic nervous
system (SoNS)—   system (ANS)—
voluntary movement   involuntary functions

sympathetic nervous
system (SNS)—
flight or fight

• increases heart rate

• inhibits digestion

• prepares lungs

• stimulates liver

• stimulates secretion of epinephrine
and norepinephrine

parasympathetic nervous
system (PSNS)—rest and digest,
feed and breed

• decreases heart rate

• stimulates digestion

• constricts lungs

• releases bile through liver

Figure 1.1 Classical AT techniques affect the ANS,
which includes the SNS and PSNS.

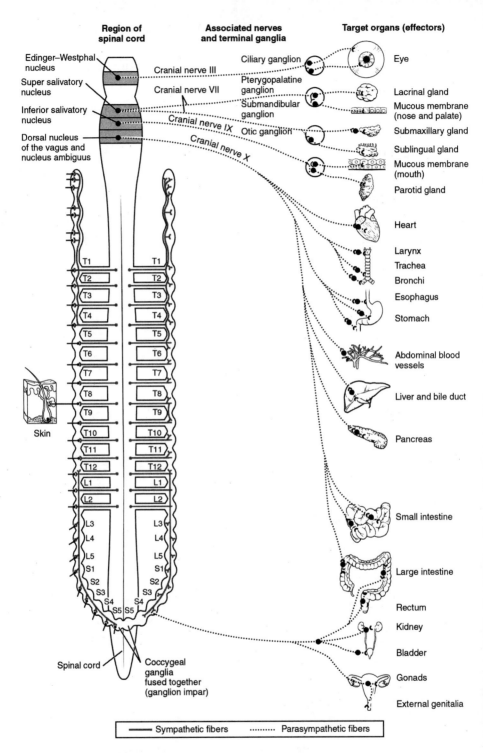

Figure 1.2. The autonomic nervous system (ANS).
From OpenStax College, 2013.

CNS overrides autonomic functioning, then our self-regulating systems break down.

WHAT AUTONOMIC TRAINING CAN DO

Classical AT is useful in changing dysfunctional autonomic functioning back to healthy operation. Heart rate, digestion, respiratory rate, sexual arousal, breathing and swallowing, blood flow—all are autonomic functions that can be self-regulated with classical AT techniques. During AT a person can augment physiological activity through practices of passive volition. This is the main difference between AT and many other mental and physiological treatments and practices wherein people actively attempt to acquire control, or a therapist controls the treatment and outcome. Popular therapist-controlled modalities include acupuncture, chiropractic, counseling, osteopathy, hypnosis, massage, psychotherapy, reflexology, shiatsu, Rolfing, and watsu, among others. Closest to AT are biofeedback (the therapist provides the machinery and instruction but the client partially controls the process), yoga (the practitioner may or may not follow a leader), and meditation (mostly practiced alone).

Johannes Schultz was first inspired by the reports of the feats of Indian yogis with regard to self-regulation of the body. However, many of the most amazing Indian yogic practices had as by-products the lack of personal responsibility, extreme poverty, and reliance on others for food and shelter. This is certainly not appropriate behavior for most modern Westerners. What Schultz found through years of clinical study was that although maybe not to the extreme of the Indian yogis it is possible for anyone to control autonomic functioning toward the goal of increased vitality and better health.

So if this is the case you may be wondering why you haven't heard of AT before. The question is fairly easy to answer in two parts. First, autogenic training takes a lot of practice. It is *training*, just like any other kind of training. You couldn't take an average person out of a crowd and say to him, "Now you are a yogi; you can self-regulate your body." Similarly, someone with no training in football could never effectively play quarterback in the Super Bowl. The truth is that most people in English-speaking countries, for whatever reasons, would rather go see some sort of therapist or doctor than try to learn how to heal themselves by themselves, through daily practices. Second, the vast majority of AT literature is currently in German, Japanese, and Russian, so is not widely available to English speakers. In Japan, AT is widely employed and very commonplace. In German-speaking countries a large portion of medical practitioners use it as an adjunct in treating various ailments.

Classical AT consists of two basic series of training exercises. The first series focuses on (1) the breathing mechanism, called *regulation;* (2) the neuromuscular system, called *the heaviness experience;* (3) the vasomotor system, called *the experience of warmth;* (4) the heart, called *regulation;* (5) warmth in the visceral organs, called *regulation;* and (6) the cooling of the forehead, called *regulation of the head.*

The second series is for those who have mastered the first series, which usually takes six to twelve months of training. It consists of exercises of passive concentration and visual imaging that at the deepest level leads to the understanding of one's own true nature. Both series and their practices will be discussed and explained further in chapters 8 and 9.

2
WHAT IS
PRIMAL MIND?

We all have the awareness of our primal mind (PM) to a certain extent. For example, we know we have to eat and drink and have shelter and warmth; we have sexual urges and the fight-or-flight mechanism. However, modern humans* have by and large forgotten many of the key aspects of primal mind awareness. One of the key, and I believe most important, aspects of primal mind awareness concerns modern people's relationship to nature. Modern humans have lost a significant portion of their primal mind awareness because we spend almost all of our time indoors, in artificially controlled environments. Most of us work in those same types of indoor environments. We send our kids to them, too, to be educated.

It is not my goal to introduce techniques of primal mind so that we can all go back to living in caves; quite the opposite. Speaking from personal experience, it is my belief that modern people can learn AT-PM techniques that will enhance modern life by waking us up to a more balanced view of ourselves and our natural environment. As German philosopher Ernst Cassirir (1874–1945), one of the leading advocates of philosophical idealism, said:

---

*To simplify I will use this term to describe people living in industrial and technological societies, the main traits being dependence on money, living in permanent buildings, reliance on grocery stores for food, etc.—in general this includes all Western societies.

What is characteristic of primal mentality is not its logic but its general sentiment of life. Primal man does not look at nature with the eyes of a naturalist who wishes to classify things in order to satisfy an intellectual curiosity. He does not approach it with merely pragmatic or technical interest. It is for him neither a mere object of knowledge nor the field of his immediate practical needs. We are in the habit of dividing our life into the two spheres of practical and theoretical activity. In this division we are prone to forget that there is . . . stratum beneath them both. Primal man is not liable to such forgetfulness. All his thoughts and his feelings are still embedded in this original stratum. His view of nature is neither merely theoretical nor merely practical; it is *sympathetic*. If we miss this point we cannot find the approach to the mystic world. Primal man by no means lacks the ability to grasp the empirical differences of things. But in his conception of nature and life all these differences are obliterated by a stronger feeling: the deep conviction of a fundamental and indelible solidarity of life that bridges over the multiplicity and variety of its single forms. He does not ascribe himself to a unique and privileged place in the scale of nature.[1]

EUROCENTRISM AND THE WESTERN VIEW OF PRIMAL PEOPLE

English naturalist and geologist Charles Robert Darwin (1809–1882) was famously known for his theory of evolution, in which he established that all life on Earth shares common descent, and that the different species are a result of an evolutionary process involving natural selection. Darwin explained that the struggle for existence through natural selection is in many ways similar to the artificial selection involved in selective breeding. He believed that he could vaguely recognize the humanlike ape as a distant cousin to *Homo sapiens*.

Darwin's theory of evolution revolutionized Western* thinking when it was introduced in the 1800s. Later, in the 1920s, Australian anthropologist Raymond Dart (1893–1988) and his colleagues unearthed an ancient "ape man" in South Africa, which Dart named *Australopithecus africanus.* The image of this carnivorous, club-swinging, bipedal ape man set the pervasive stereotype of our ancient ancestors for future generations of not only scientists but lay people as well. The cruel and bloodthirsty ape man came to be looked at as the quintessential opposite of the prevalent Victorian† concept of what civilization represents.

From there it was quite natural for Westerners to figure the so-called ape man as the earliest stage of human evolution, while arranging in a vertical series of developments the position of the white Victorian male at the summit of human evolution. This Eurocentric viewpoint had an important impact on those people and cultures encountered through Western imperialism and colonization, where non-Europeans were often simply regarded as nothing more than barbaric pagans. American writer and journalist Jamake Highwater says, "This consensus established a highly ethnocentric anthropological error: the farther back in the 'ancestral cave' you live the more 'primitive' you are and, therefore, the more lowly by comparison to the white male, who places himself at the crown of creation. It is immediately clear how readily this error has served the political and economic aggressiveness of the West."[2] And although it is clear that modern scientists now have a very

---

*Western civilization or culture broadly refers to the social norms, ethical values, traditional customs, belief systems, political systems, and specific artifacts and technologies that have some origin or association with Europe. The term *Western* in reality refers to technological advancement, in contrast to *non-Western,* which is essentially a euphemism for "primitive," designating any society that falls outside of Europe or areas historically colonized by Europe.

†The largely peaceful and prosperous Victorian era of British history occurred during the period of Queen Victoria's reign, from June 20, 1837, until her death on January 22, 1901. During Victoria's era the British Empire sought to colonize the far-off lands of nonwhite peoples. Culturally, Victorianism was characterized by straight-laced morality and the refined manners of European civilization.

different view of our distant ancestors, the fact remains that Westerners still, whether consciously or subconsciously, tend to measure all things against our dominant Eurocentric society. From the Western viewpoint, the less European your facial structure, skin color, and other physical traits, the less "civilized" your art and culture is considered, and therefore the lower your status, which makes you easier to exploit.

The Eurocentric outlook is perhaps best epitomized in the works of Turgot (1727–1781), a French economist and statesman who was educated at the theological college of the Sorbonne in Paris and is noted for two Latin dissertations, *On the Benefits which the Christian Religion has conferred on Mankind,* and *On the Historical Progress of the Human Mind.* Turgot believed firmly that progress is the most important factor in human evolution. Progress, according to Turgot, meant agriculture and domestication of animals so one didn't have to spend all one's waking hours searching for food. Progress freed up time for building churches and houses and created leisure time for creations of music, art, and writing. In Turgot's way of thinking, primal people were engaged in a 24/7, 365-days-a-year battle for simple survival, and as such they had no free time to progress from their pitiful lives.

Of course, we now know that the assumption that primal people had and have no free time is erroneous. Modern studies show that people in surviving primal cultures have in fact much more free time than the average Westerner. I have experienced this myself in my time living with the Huichol and other primal cultures. The Huichol work very long, hard hours during certain times of year when they plant and harvest their corn. However, the other times of the year they are very relaxed, and there is much time for personal pursuits such as weaving, making art, traveling, and making music. The Eurocentric bias so prevalent in our world today is a situation I hope will change one day, especially in consideration of my Native American friends who live "out of sight, out of mind," far from their ancestral homelands, in shacks on reservations.

Nicolas de Condorcet, a philosopher and political scientist of the 1700s, was another influential Eurocentrist. Condorcet took Turgot's philosophies and beliefs a step further with regard to distinguishing primal peoples and Western culture. He proposed the idea that a culture's evolutionary status could be judged according to the achievements of Western civilization. He believed that there is only one path to human evolution, and that all people must take this same path in order to progress to the high level of Western civilization. All other paths that do not lead toward the progress achieved by the West he considered backward and irrelevant.

The ideas of evolutionary progress advocated by Turgot and Condorcet (which linger even to this day) were supported by the evaluations of primal peoples by Charles de Brosses (1709–1777), a French writer and "scholar of evolution." De Brosses* classified primal cultures as childish due mostly to their rituals and ceremonies related to animal hunting. But worse than merely seeing primal people as acting like children, de Brosses asserted that Western children most naturally, and due to the high advancements of Western culture, mature into highly productive adults, whereas primal people live their whole life in perpetual infancy.

ROMANTICISM AND THE IDEALIZATION OF PRIMAL PEOPLES

A positive outcome as relates to our discussion, with implications for both the French Revolution and the American Revolutionary War, was that around this time many other scholars and philosophers began to question the ambitions of Western civilization. With the incomprehensible suffering and loss of life that came with revolution and war, people started to ponder ideals of progress and industry as primary human concerns; this gave birth to Romanticism. Some of the characteristic attitudes of the Romantic period, which occurred approximately during the first half of the nineteenth century, were a deepened appreciation of

---

*De Brosses was an enemy of the famous Enlightenment writer and polygenist Voltaire, who apparently barred de Brosses's entry to the Académie Française in 1770.

the beauties of nature; a general exaltation of emotion over reason, and of the senses over intellect; introspection and a heightened examination of human personality and its moods and mental potentialities; an emphasis on imagination as a gateway to transcendent experience and spiritual truth; an obsessive interest in folk culture and national and ethnic cultural origins; and a predilection, if not idealization, of the exotic, the remote, the mysterious, the weird, the occult, the monstrous, the diseased, and even the satanic.

As part of its reassessment of the rationalism of the Enlightenment, the Romantic era also ushered in a new and enhanced study of primal cultures. As an outcome of this, many romanticists started describing primal cultures in a way previously unheard of and considered profane by strict rationalists. Unspoiled by the atrocities of Western civilization and the church, primal peoples were portrayed by the Romantics as naturally good, living without greed for material possessions, and to have a healthy, symbiotic relationship with nature.

With the emergence of the writings of transcendentalist Henry David Thoreau (1817–1862) and through the influence of Leo Tolstoy (1828–1910) and geographer Élisée Reclus (1830–1905), among others, anarchist-naturism appeared as the union of anarchist and naturist philosophies. This hybrid philosophy of life was in direct contrast to the views of Turgot and others of his ilk. Anarcho-naturism promoted an ecological worldview, small ecovillages, and even nudism as a way to avoid the artificiality of industrial culture. Naturist-individualist anarchists saw the individual in his or her biological, physical, and psychological aspects and avoided and tried to eliminate social determinations.

Today, anarcho-primitivism* is gaining popularity as more and more people are becoming disillusioned by our technological society. Anarcho-primitivism is an anarchist critique of the origins and so-called progress of Western civilization. According to anarcho-primitivism, the shift from hunter-gatherer to agricultural subsistence gave rise to

---

*Anarcho-primitivists tend to not like being tagged by one word, but currently it's the most accurate one we have to describe them.

social stratification, coercion, alienation, and extreme population growth. Anarcho-primitivists advocate a return to "noncivilized" ways of life through deindustrialization, abolition of the division of labor or specialization, and the abandonment of large-scale organizational technologies.

The Romantic Era only lasted about five decades and was replaced by science-based philosophies that disregarded any nonindustrialized, non-Western peoples. And so primal peoples were once again relegated to a position of ambiguity. On the American continents, anthropologists* and missionaries pursued a Eurocentric agenda in trying to comprehend the startling occurrence of ancient civilizations discovered as a result of the "discovery" of the so-called New World.

CHRISTIAN ETHNOGRAPHY AND "SCIENTIFIC RACISM"

In a way it is quite comical, but in the end just plain sad, that we still hold on to the single collective term *Indian* to describe people who never used a single name to describe the vast number of different and unique tribes living on this continent and offshore islands. And they certainly weren't Indian. The mistake of Columbus, that he had found a shortcut to the East Indies, is well documented.† He called the native inhabitants of this continent *Indians* because that's where he thought he actually was! We really can't blame the directionally challenged Columbus for the term. It is much more interesting that even after much debate as to the origins of aboriginal Americans, and after geographical proof of

---

*Many scholars consider modern anthropology an outgrowth of the Age of Enlightenment (approximately 1650–1780), a period when Europeans attempted to study the cultures of the "other" systematically.
†During his homeward voyage, Columbus penned a letter to the royal court in Barcelona. In this letter he makes six references to India or the Indies, and four to the inhabitants, which he called *Indios*. The letter rapidly became a fifteenth-century best seller throughout Western Europe, with no fewer than eleven editions produced in 1493 in Spain, Italy, France, Switzerland, and the Netherlands.

the existence of the Western Hemisphere, the use of the word *Indian* continued, as it does to this day.

The European explorers—or invaders, depending on your point of view—quickly realized Columbus's discovery was not a part of Asia but an entirely "New World" filled with people and flora and fauna unknown to them. Since Christian clergymen almost always traveled with the European explorers to begin the process of colonization, a major question immediately formed in the minds of Europeans: How was it possible that these people existed when they were not mentioned in the Scriptures or in Genesis, in the biblical story of the Creation? What about the children of Noah repopulating the world after the Great Flood? There's really no mention of them there either. These were questions that plagued the minds of the Christian theologians. The biggest question ultimately cropped up: were these people even human? Since the Bible recounts that God created humanity in a single act, then they must be human. But how could their existence be traced back to Adam and Eve? The vast differences in language, skin color, lifestyle, and technology, among many other things, confounded orthodox Christians of the time. The church fathers needed a biblical explanation, and what they came up with was found in Genesis 11:4–9. The story goes like this:

After the Great Flood, everyone on Earth spoke the same language. As people migrated outward from the east, they settled in the land of Shinar. People there sought to make bricks and build a city and a tower (the famous Tower of Babel) with its top in the sky. God looked at the city and the tower and considered this act hubristic. He remarked that as one people with one language, nothing that they sought would be out of their reach, such that they would become competitors of God Himself. Therefore, God scrambled their speech so that they couldn't understand one another, scattering them over the face of the earth so that they stopped building the city. Thus the city was called Babel, from the Hebrew word *balal,* meaning "to jumble." So the short Christian explanation is that Native Americans originally came to North and

South America as a result of the dispersion of people at the time of the Tower of Babel.

But the Church Fathers still had a nagging problem. How could these heathens of the New World be so different in almost every way from the Europeans who had discovered them? To answer this question, the Christian ideologues postulated the idea of degeneration: after the dispersion and the abandonment of Babel, some of humankind degenerated and declined into idolatry and heathenism, and wide differences in language, customs, and manners combined as the decay of peoples' ability to grasp the knowledge of the One True God continued. In this view, Indians were viewed as simply corrupted Jews from the biblical past.

In the late 1800s, science began to overtake Christian ethnography in terms of influence, and a new "science of race" was postulated. This updated approach attempted to explain racial differences with a comprehensive study of human anatomy. One of the featured methods of this new science was conducted by Samuel George Morton (1799–1851), an American physician and natural scientist. Morton is often considered the originator of the so-called American school of ethnography that arose during the slavery era of the United States. This dubious branch of science—really pseudoscience—claimed the difference between humans was one of species rather than variety; in fact, it is widely regarded as the origin of and justification for racism. Morton argued against the simple Creation story of the Bible (monogenism) and instead supported a theory of multiple racial creations (polygenism). He claimed the Bible supported polygenism, and within working in a biblical framework, his theory held that each race had been created separately, and each was given specific, irrevocable characteristics.

To prove this, Morton popularized the cephalic index, or cranial index: the ratio of the maximum width of the head of an organism (human or animal) multiplied by 100, divided by its maximum length. Morton claimed that through this method of craniometry he could define the intellectual ability of a race by skull capacity. A large volume meant a large brain and high intellectual capacity, and a small skull indicated a small brain and decreased intellectual capacity. Among humans he (naturally) assigned the highest brain capacity to Europeans, with the English highest of all, followed by Chinese, Southeast Asians and Polynesians, and in fourth place, American Indians. The smallest brain capacity was assigned to Africans and Australian aborigines. These measurements were seen by Morton to prove conclusively the superiority of whites over all other races. The "scientific racism" of this time period reasoned that it was no accident that white men developed the highest civilization known to mankind and ruled the world; it was simply biological inheritance that made them superior, and nonwhites irreversibly inferior.[3] Although Morton was nominally a scientist, he used his influence to make the case for black inferiority in order to bolster U.S. Secretary of State John Calhoun's efforts to negotiate the annexation of Texas as a slave state.

Then in the late 1800s and early 1900s the field of psychology emerged. This newest scientific discipline generally supported racial differences insofar as primal people were thought to be instinct-driven (a feature common to animals), and only highly advanced cultures such as Europeans could create literature, complex music and art, and democratic government. During this time period, science, this time in the form of psychology, once again categorized primal peoples as inferior to Europeanized Westerners. However, this kind of thinking didn't last too long, and by the mid-1900s the social sciences discredited blatant racism and replaced it with ideals of cultural pluralism.* But political and economic racism endured, as it still does today, as the dominant society continued to subjugate certain peoples and races for monetary gain and civic power. In recent times in the United States, as people have become more and more distrustful and oftentimes clearly angry

---

*In a pluralist culture, unique groups not only coexist side by side but also consider qualities of other groups as traits worth having in the dominant culture. A successful pluralistic society will place strong expectations of integration on its members rather than expectations of assimilation.

with organized religion, it has become quite fashionable for white people to explore and even appropriate Native American spirituality. Two of the most popular sites of these kinds of explorations are the Hopi and Navaho lands. There are literally thousands of books that have been written for Western people about the practices of native spirituality, and hundreds of courses, workshops, and retreats that teach white people about native traditions. One of the most popular current trends is for Western people to travel to South America to visit primal shamans to ingest the plant entheogen ayahuasca for psychological healing and enlightenment.

PRESENT-DAY SITES OF PRIMAL MIND

The place of primal people in the Western mind continues to fluctuate between directions offered by science, spirituality, and humanism. My descriptions and techniques of primal mind in this book are not formulated to undermine Western mentality but to bring to light an alternative view that has been disparaged, cast out, and neglected for centuries— just as gays, females, and nonwhites have been abused within white male Western culture. From my point of view the Lakota phrase *Mitakuye Oyasin* is appropriate when exploring the mind of primal people in relation to Western thought. The phrase translates as "all my relatives," "we are all related," or "all my relations." It is a prayer of oneness and harmony with all forms of life: other people as well as animals, birds, insects, trees and other plants, and even rocks, rivers, mountains, and valleys. "We are all related" is an affirmation of the metaphysical truth of the interconnection of all life, including humans. As the renowned psychiatrist Carl Jung, who traveled widely as a student of "primitive" psychology, so eloquently stated, "We all finally unite in one family tree, but what is a tree without its elaborately dissimilar branches?"[4]

There still exist large areas and small niches of the world where people manage to live totally or partially with primal mind as the dominant portion of their identity and activities. These are the peoples who for one reason or another have avoided being converted into the two most prevalent evangelistic religions, Christianity and Islam. They also, by and large, do not participate in the global industrial-technological economy and live "off the grid." In terms of geography this is an overview of those cultures:

- Africa is a continent that contains areas that have been subjected to wide-scale human-rights abuses of the worst kind as a result of European colonization over many centuries. Nevertheless, there are still large areas that have managed to remain primal.
- Most ancient European native traditions are well documented; some of these pagan traditions continue to remain viable for people even today.
- Northern Siberia's native traditions have remained intact longer than elsewhere in the Russian Federation, in part because the land there is less economically desirable than other places in modern times.
- China has been recovering from an identity crisis stemming from the British Opium Wars in the nineteenth century; since then its government has taken varying stands on the status of native spirituality. However, there are still over fifty indigenous groups that hold to their ancient customs.
- India has legal protections in place since the mid-twentieth century for what are called "scheduled tribes," "scheduled castes," and "other backward classes."
- Middle Eastern native traditions are documented in various ways. A great tragedy of the twenty-first century was the loss of Mesopotamian religious artifacts in the American-instigated Iraqi War. The Middle East is now flooded with modern technology, goods, and weapons, but there remain areas where primal awareness is still prevalent.
- Pacific Island tribal spiritual traditions and language are some of the best preserved and are still practiced by the Maori and other

native Pacific Islanders, including native Hawaiians, as witnessed by the current Hawaiian sovereignty movement.

- When the Americas were "discovered" by Westerners in the late fifteenth century, they were actually already inhabited in most viable regions. Very few indigenous peoples north of Mexico now live without thorough or partial integration into nonindigenous society. Nevertheless, in Central and South America, and in isolated areas of North America, there exist pockets of primal people who still practice their native lifeways to this day.

The last group on this list is where my own understanding of primal mind derives from. For over twenty-five years I have lived among and experienced the primal-mind awareness of the Huichol and other native tribes north and south of the U.S. border with Mexico. In my previous book, *Teachings of the Peyote Shamans,* I detailed my personal experiences with the amazing Huichol people. I wrote *The Flying Witches of Veracruz* about what I learned from living with an indigenous group in the jungle of eastern Mexico, and in my book *Lightning in My Blood* I shared twenty-three stories of fascinating lessons taught to me by primal elders of the Seneca, Lenni Lenape, Apurimac Inca, Arapaho, Minnecojou Sioux, Kanaka Maoli, Tuscarora, Tukano, Mazatek, Yurok, Navaho, Hopi, Yucatec Maya, and Huichol/Wirrarika.

In terms of religion, primal cultures are generally henotheistic; that is, they believe in one single Creator god while acknowledging the existence of other gods. In this view, God dwells within all things, and all things are spiritual in nature. All of existence is thought to be interconnected, including life and death, humans and animals, the physical world and the spirit world. Primal cultures do not discern between the physical and the spiritual, nor is there a hard distinction between worship and other day-to-day activities of life. Living in and of itself is a spiritual act; the duties of each day are so intertwined with nature and the earth that they are regarded as spiritual, as opposed to compartmentalizing life into work, leisure, and worship. The primal concept of time is also different; time is not linear, as Western cultures think of it, and instead the idea of timelessness is widely accepted. Rituals are enacted as performances of the original act of Creation and are ever present and thus link individuals to eternity through the present.

Although this is radically changing in many areas of the world, primal cultures are generally preliterate and lack written language. Their beliefs and traditions are orally disseminated, usually through stories, songs, and art. These modalities of expression are passed down through the generations to explain the origins of humans, the nature of God, and explanations of the world's workings. Most often these stories, songs, and art forms are tied to the region in which they are experienced, as people are closely tied to the earth and the locale in which they live.

Rites of passage are of great importance in these societies, as is the concept of liminality, the state of transition between various rites of passage. Rites of passage are distinguished by rituals, which play a large role in tribal life. The tribe, which extends beyond just persons to include nature, animals, and objects both animate and inanimate, is central to the individual's sense of self. In this sense the infusion of autogenic training and primal mind awareness into a modern person's life could be seen as a powerful rite of passage.

THE PRIMAL "MINDSCAPE"

One of the most significant lessons I have learned through my experiences with primal elders is the ability to travel in a different kind of landscape, one characterized by altered states of consciousness intentionally induced in order to tap into the vast knowledge and power of the universe beyond human thoughts or concepts. In this state the world is experienced without written words and without preconceived opinions or biases. There is no division between inner and outer, and reality is perceived beyond the normal constructs of time and space. It is not some sort of obscure esoteric or supernatural state but rather a heightening of our experience of reality.

As an illustration of this idea and how it relates to PM techniques, I will delineate human consciousness so as to explain the marked differences between the various levels:

1. This first level of consciousness I refer to as ordinary for our modern culture and for other cultures that have lost a sense of unity with nature and the cosmos. At this level the ego is almost completely self-centered and isolated from the occurrences of the more-than-human world.

2. On the second level there is a slight awareness of fusion between the self and the surrounding environment of nature and other beings. Because of this the capacity for empathy manifests, but not at a level that would prevent people from doing harm or damage to something or someone outside their narrow sphere of compassion if they deemed it was called for.

3. At the third level we see the first signs of the ego temporarily melding with the environment or with other beings. This often occurs briefly during moments of being in natural environments of extreme beauty or when witnessing wild animals in their natural habitats.

4. The fourth level is significant for primal mind because here we identify our human organism with a much larger unified body—with plants and animals, and with other phenomena and forms of communication not accessible at the lower levels. We can experience consciousness free of human evaluations and judgments, even if for only a short time.

5. At the fifth level of consciousness the feeling of unity between self and one's environment leads to experiences of "silent knowledge," telepathy, the ability to transfer energy or heal, compress or lengthen the perception of time, and other circumstances commonly thought to be supernatural or extrasensory. At this level many experiences simply cannot be explained by words.

6. The sixth level is the level free from all human attachments, as if your personal organism and consciousness were completely non-discernable from the unified consciousness of the cosmos.

In terms of this delineation we could say that in general primal mind happens within levels 3, 4, and 5. I would add that PM is stimulated by participation in the natural world, whether intentional or not. In other words, at each level an experience of unity with the natural world stimulates the shift to a deeper, more profound connection to the environment and the corresponding loss of attachment to purely human concerns. Through intentionally practicing PM awareness and purposefully struggling through various actions, techniques, and rituals with the more-than-human world, a person realizes increasing states of unity; first with others of her own kind and her immediate environment, then with other beings and the wider world, and eventually with powers and forces inconceivable in the linear-rational mode of perception.

Some of the most important aspects of primal mind awareness as a modern-day rite of passage include experiences of learning from a source of knowledge much larger than the confines of strictly human affairs. Visions, intuition, perception of sentience in plants, and communication with animals are common PM experiences. PM awareness also brings the experience of death and rebirth. Dismemberment, dissolving, exploding, and other experiences of being killed and then reborn into a stronger and healthier state, although seemingly traumatizing, can be truly enlightening and empowering experiences. PM experiences can be heightened by music, singing, chanting, dancing, drumming, and other nonintellectual activities that enhance the flow of the experience. PM awareness brings the perception of Spirit. This may come in many forms, but throughout this book are many practices of AT-PM that invoke feelings of a Higher Power and connection to the spirit of nature.

All of these intentional experiences have one goal: to help balance our psychophysiological organism through the introduction of lost forms of primal mind that raise our consciousness.

3

COMBINING AUTOGENIC TRAINING AND PRIMAL MIND AWARENESS

Now that we've taken a look at both AT and PM, it's time to put them together. Why? Because each on its own is incomplete in terms of the desired outcome. AT takes us deeper inside our physiology, while PM informs us of how we relate to the world and how the world relates to us. Techniques that bring the two together have the power of true transformation. With the tool of classical AT it is possible to enter deep states of PM and rediscover moments of psychophysiological homeostasis, a balance between mind, body, the natural world, and the spirit of all things. By adding primal mind awareness to classical autogenic techniques, we now discover a new way to create balance in our lives. That is the goal of this book.

AT-PM practices produce altered states of consciousness. In this respect we may generally say that an AT-PM technique that produces an altered state is one that disrupts the normal stream of thoughts by producing a new rhythm or quality of psychophysiological awareness. Table 3.1 (pages 28–29) shows examples of our ordinary states and those acquired during or after practicing AT-PM techniques.

TABLE 3.1. ORDINARY STATE VERSUS ALTERED STATE

Aspect of Ordinary State in Daily Life in the Modern World	Aspect of Altered State during or after AT-PM Practices
We feel at various levels the existential void and loneliness of being an autonomous, independent entity.	The world and universe are perceived as a unified whole, and we not only are part of this whole, we have an integral place and niche within it.
Personal consciousness is limited to the boundaries of the physical body; e.g., the head or brain.	A melding of primal consciousness occurs between the practitioner and other entities such as plants, animals, trees, and elements.
We automatically evaluate, compare, and judge the people, places, and things around us.	Attention and concentration are intentionally focused in passive ways that foster a connection with other life forms and energies at a level that doesn't judge, evaluate, or compare. Everything that we perceive is accepted as equally important and awesome.
Pride is often a self-inflating emotion or response to a chaotic world, a kind of machismo that is not often associated with humility or humbleness.	A transcendental feeling of unity allows a person to be proud and humble at the same time.
We perceive the world relative to human beings. The world is here for us to use, and the majority of our time is spent on our purely self-centered, human concerns.	The world is perceived in a much larger context than strictly human concerns. Human beings are but one voice in a grand chorus.
We are in a continuous search to find meaning and value in our actions and for our life.	The experience is felt as having intrinsic value, and many times the experience touches our primal soul so deeply that it provides real meaning and value to our life.
We are consciously in touch with the passage of time by very frequently checking our watch or clock or calendar to see what time it is and where we are at on that linear continuum.	Significant alterations in the perception of time occur. It is common for a moment to feel like a lifetime or a day to feel like an hour.
Because of all of the perceived and manufactured crises of modern times we often get stuck dwelling on the problems of the world and of our personal lives.	It is more common than not to experience the world as beautiful, magnificent, and meaningful. Positive and negative, good and evil are equally accepted as part of the greater whole. This most often leads to focusing attention and action on that which makes life valuable and worthwhile.

Aspect of Ordinary State in Daily Life in the Modern World	Aspect of Altered State during or after AT-PM Practices
Our actions are often aggressive in order to succeed. We tend to miss a lot by rushing around to accomplish tasks.	The capacity to receive, as in sensing, feeling, and listening, is enhanced through a more passive and humble state of being.
Much of the everyday feelings associated with the sacred or divine are lost through our hectic, fast-paced lives.	Feelings such as awe, humbleness, wonder, mystery, reverence, and sacredness are experienced.
We tend to view death as tragic, we do everything we can to avoid it, and we often go to our graves with feelings of resentment for our life having been taken away. This cultural view of death tends to make us more aggressive and belligerent during life.	A peaceful acceptance of death as one of life's many changes is commonly felt. This fosters a deep, primal feeling of harmony with the world during life.
We feel like we know more than what we don't know. Mechanistic, materialistic views attempt to reduce everything to what is known empirically.	We awaken to the fact that there is so much more that we don't know than what we do know. Mystery is embraced as we humbly acknowledge that some things may be forever unknowable.
We are often trapped by feelings of inadequacy, anxiety, and confusion. Our life path is commonly guided by society and authority figures rather than the unfolding of our life occurring naturally and spontaneously.	Experiences of awe and unity give a person increased ability to transcend his or her perceived limitations. A renewed confidence is felt so that daily life is more self-directed toward an authentic calling in life.
Our earthly existence is normally felt as being subordinate to what might be described as heaven.	It is common to feel that heaven is what you make of it here on Earth during life.
The modern world often creates very callous and malicious people.	People are often described by others as more loving, accepting, kind, compassionate, and less selfish.
People tend to dwell on the negative. "If it weren't for bad luck I'd have no luck at all."	People tend to feel more "in the flow"— blessed, lucky, and fortunate.
We are accustomed to solving life problems chiefly through personal thoughts and human knowledge.	It's common to receive messages and visions pertinent to our life situations from beings and entities that we normally don't communicate with.

Table expanded and revised from *Ecoshamanism: Sacred Practices of Unity, Power and Earth Healing,* by James Endredy

Obviously, this table is designed to list the positive aspects of the AT-PM experience and not the positive aspects of the modern world, of which there are, of course, many. But please keep in mind that at the deepest or highest levels the states of consciousness that AT-PM supply defy explanations with words, or at least the words of the modern English language, so many aspects of altered states cannot be included in this table. The techniques presented in this book will help you to successfully accomplish the right side of the table. From then on it is my hope that you will explore your own new and as yet uncharted techniques and share them with others (including me!).

THE EFFECTS OF AT-PM

Our initial goals for AT-PM in the experiential portion of this book can be divided into four main areas: body, mind, environment, and spirit.

Body

Realize that through AT we can control the physiological aspects of our body that are not presently known to us. We can reclaim the awareness that our physical body is the most obvious and intimate component of the natural world that we could ever know, and realize that alienating ourselves from our body also alienates us from nature. Given this truth, we realize that our physical health is continually impacted by the health or sickness of our environment and also by what our body receives as sustenance. Through AT-PM we can reconnect with the inherited ancient wisdom held within our human body. We learn that our body is capable of an awareness that is distinguishable from but complementary with the awareness of our mind.

Mind

Through experiences of primal mind we dispel the illusion that the human psyche is somehow separate from the natural world by acknowledging and granting psychological status to our relationship with the natural world. We overcome our deficient childhood psychological development, which stemmed from insufficient reciprocal and harmonious relationships with the natural world. We identify specific psychological imbalances in our relationship to the natural world and bring to light our current valuation of and affiliation with the natural world so as to critically assess both our lifestyles and our philosophical views.

Environment

Through experiences of AT-PM we recover the moment-to-moment awareness that every one of our thoughts and actions is tied to the web of life that encompasses the entire planet. As a result, we develop a deep and genuine connection with the land where we live. We learn to see a deeper reality by removing the facades and disguises that obscure the true identity of objects, situations, and circumstances.

Spirit

When we engage in AT-PM practices the controlling aspects of our ego dissolve and our consciousness flows outward in connection with the sacred elements and entities of the natural world: air, water, sun, fire, Earth, moon, as well as the animating spirits of trees, birds, animals, insects, and flowers. We develop a spiritual connection to the natural world that allows us to listen to and understand what the earth and her living entities are telling us. This allows us to find our individual reconciliation with nature's cycles of life, death, and rebirth. We create and utilize rites of passage and initiation in order to grow into wise, mature members of the earth community.

༉

PART TWO

Autogenic Training Techniques

4
PREPARING FOR AUTOGENIC TRAINING

The original format of AT as developed by Johann Heinrich Schultz consists of a series of six progressive training exercises in the first stage and an additional seven exercises that compose the advanced stage. I have supplemented* these teachings based on my own personal experiences with AT and have also incorporated feedback from participants in my workshops. Once learned, AT can be practiced anywhere, but in the beginning I recommend completing the first seven trainings with these suggestions in mind:

- Practice alone in a setting that is warm, quiet, and dimly lit. You want to be comfortable and in a place with as little possibility for interruption as possible.
- Wear comfy clothes and no shoes.
- Keep your eyes closed while practicing. If you need to make notes for yourself or remember the material it's okay to open your eyes to read the instructions; just close your eyes again while you practice.
- It can help the initial training to lie flat on your back on a hard, carpeted floor or rug. This will enhance your ability to feel the

---

*I have added the *I breathe me* formula to the basic six of Schultz because it is so important; thus, I present seven exercises in the first stage.

heaviness of your arms and legs. If that is not practical for you a bed, couch, or exercise or yoga mat will do fine. After you have mastered the complete training sequence you can use your autogenic formulas under any other circumstances you like, whether sitting, standing, walking, or lying down.

- Make sure your bladder and bowels are empty.
- It's best to practice before meals.
- Avoid intoxicants and smoking beforehand.
- If you fall asleep during a session, repeat that routine in your next session.
- If you practice in bed at night, you could fall asleep before you complete your cycle. Therefore, if you practice at night, in bed, consider this to be in addition to your basic practice.

Initially it is recommended that you practice three times a day, spread out throughout your daily schedule. This takes more discipline for some people than for others. For those of you who may feel guilty by spending your time this way just remember that you deserve it! Give yourself permission to give back to yourself. Practicing AT in the morning can help you begin your day without tension and help put you in a relaxed and peaceful state that you can maintain for the whole day. Sometimes you may feel like going back to sleep after your morning practice. If this happens to you frequently, simply add this affirmation to the current formula you are working on during your practice: "I am fully awake and focused while training."

A systematic, precise training program can bring you the most powerful results and enhance the benefits of AT. It is recommended that you set up an exact time schedule for practicing AT, particularly if you are starting the first stage sequence of seven trainings. The beginner should then follow this schedule as closely as possible.

You will discover for yourself the best time(s) to practice AT. Most people do their last exercise shortly before they go to sleep. This has many advantages, particularly for people who suffer from insomnia or have a hard time going to sleep. Unless engaged in rigorous physical activity during the day I often have problems "shutting down" my mind when it's time to sleep. The relaxation of AT quite frequently helps me stop my rambling thoughts and promotes a healthy entrance into the slumber mode. Most clients report that their morning and evening sessions are the most productive.

The midday practice is also valuable because it breaks up the day, but it is often the most challenging to accomplish, especially if you are at work. However, with enough intention it is usually possible to find a reasonably quiet place. If it's not possible to find the perfect spot, improvise. I have had trainees who work nine to five in an office setting tell me they use the restroom during their lunch break. Granted, you might not get much out of those sessions initially. But at this foundational stage we are most concerned with disciplining ourselves to follow a new routine.

As previously mentioned, the ideal setting is a quiet, dim, warm environment where you can lie still and not be disturbed. But this is not always possible, and once the practice is mastered it is not necessary. Here is a description of the standard lying-down position, followed by a description of the most effective seated body positions for learning AT:

Reclining Position

Lie on your back with your legs outstretched and slightly apart, with your feet relaxed, falling slightly outward. Your arms are at your sides, slightly away from your torso, palms facing down. An alternative position is to rest your downturned hands on either side of your pelvis. The main thing is to be comfortable. A pillow placed under your head or under your knees might be helpful. Keep your head and neck straight. Do not have any constricting sheets, covers, or clothes on you. It is not advisable when learning AT to roll on your side, as when going to sleep.

Meditative Position

You can practice AT (or meditate—see chapter 9) in a public place using a chair (or even in the restroom, using the toilet as a chair). It's fine to simply sit with your back comfortably resting against the back of the chair (or if there's no chair back, simply sit up straight), with your neck in a straight line with your spine. If using a seated position the feet should be flat on the floor, with the angle of your knees to your feet greater than 90 degrees so that your feet are out in front of you. (If your knees are at 90 degrees or less, with your feet under your thighs, your feet can easily fall asleep and disrupt your practice.)

Easy-Chair Position

As this implies, you use an easy chair or even a couch with pillows for supporting your back and neck. However, make sure your feet are flat on the floor with your knees at a greater-than 90-degree angle in front of you.

Rag-Doll Position

Sit in a chair without armrests. Get into the meditative posture described above and then scoot toward the front of the chair so the backs of your legs are not touching the chair, feet flat on the floor and knees bent at a greater-than 90-degree angle in front of you. Spread your feet slightly wider than normal. Now let your arms hang loosely at your sides and then stretch your spine and neck up high toward the ceiling so that you are comfortable in this erect posture. Now imagine there is an elastic cord attached to the crown of your head that is connected to the ceiling. Let the cord snap, allowing your neck and back to relax into a gentle curve. This should be a comfortable position, yet with your chest not so caved-in as to inhibit full breathing. Finally, rest your hands in your lap, palms down.

Now it is important to introduce what is called the *cancellation*. Please pay careful attention to this, as we will be using this in every AT session. When you are finished with an exercise it is best to end your session in a way that will return you to your normal state, awake and alert. You may in time come up with your own method for doing this. Here's the recommended way to start:

Canceling an AT Session

Open your fingers by strongly stretching them. Bend your elbows so that your forearms form a right angle with your chest. Take a deep breath while at the same time bringing your hands together in a prayer position, with the sides of your thumbs firmly resting against your chest. Exhale deeply while extending your arms out in front of you,* allowing your hands to separate, palms still facing each other. Open your eyes. This can be done once or as many times as needed until you feel fully alert.

Before explaining the exercises I want to reiterate what I mean by passive volition, the most important aspect of AT. As explained in chapter 1, passive volition involves planting a seed in your mind and simply letting it grow in your subconscious and throughout your body, without worrying it to death. Although this may seem simple, in terms of human concentration and the way we have been taught to use our attention, this can take some time to learn. Don't be discouraged if you don't get it right away. If you keep to your training schedule you will realize passive volition, and it will become your best friend.

Since it is not unusual to perhaps want to try all the techniques at once, or rush through them, I have laid out the beginning sessions in a day-by-day format to better ensure success. I suggest you try this format and not proceed to the next training exercise until you feel confident in the previous one.

---

*In most cases this is done gently at the end of a series or session, but if you need to cancel a session immediately, for whatever reason, you can do so more forcefully by throwing your arms out strongly and exhaling powerfully.

5
THE SEVEN STANDARD FORMULAS

Training #1
Breathing—The *I Breathe Me* Experience

The first training, *I Breathe Me,* is so simple that on the surface it might seem too obvious; but as you get inside this exercise and go deeper you will understand how important it is to the whole series. The importance of the first training with our breath sets the stage for passive volition, the cornerstone of autogenic training.

There are many relaxation, healing, and meditative techniques that employ altering one's breath in one way or another, and they are quite effective. But in AT we do just the opposite: we try to do nothing at all with our breathing. Breathing is an autonomous activity of the body that we know we can control so it is the perfect activity to begin learning AT and, more specifically, passive volition. In AT it is undesirable to alter one's breathing intentionally, since we want to self-regulate our body through *passive* volition, not active adjustment. During AT the muscular and vascular systems naturally integrate with our breathing.

In this training we try to do nothing at all with our breathing, and so we use the passive-sounding statement *I breathe me.* This statement makes it clear that regulation of the breath will come naturally and spontaneously during the training. We use this phrase while concentrating not on the rising and falling movement of the chest, but rather on the air that comes in and out of the nose or mouth. Inhale through the nose and exhale either through the nose or mouth—whichever feels more comfortable. In a comfortable AT position, focusing on the breath without trying to alter it, we can enter the deep state of relaxation that is passive volition and thereby prepare for the other trainings.

It is recommended that you do this training many times during your first day. Since it is the first step to all the other trainings, it's important to take your time and get used to it.

Begin when ready:

+ Get into a comfortable AT position, either reclining or seated, as described in the previous chapter, although if you are new to the training it can help to lie flat on your back on a rug or carpet on a hard floor.
+ Concentrate on the breath coming in and out of your nose and mouth without trying to regulate it; just let it flow easily, in and out, while slowly and silently repeating the phrase *I breathe me.* Do not vocalize the phrase; simply hear it in your mind. It is not necessary to repeat the phrase on each breath because it becomes too repetitious. I usually say it on each breath for the first few breaths, and then after that, maybe every three or four breaths, whatever feels comfortable and natural for you. Do this for a minimum of two minutes or for as long as you wish.
+ Cancel.

Training #2
Neuromuscular System—The Heaviness Experience

This second training is based on the neuromuscular system, the integrated efforts of both the nervous and the muscular systems. It tends to be the second-easiest system influenced by conscious efforts, and it also provides a concrete set of practices that results in a deep level of relaxation. There are many ways to relax muscles. Two of my favorites are soaking in geothermal hot springs and massage. However, the goal here is to self-generate muscular relaxation. We begin our AT training very methodically, by first concentrating on only our dominant arm on day one. Then throughout the week we add the other arm and eventually both legs. It wouldn't be useful in the beginning to attempt training that encompasses the whole body before we learn how to do it with specific body parts and bodily functions. However, if successful training has been accomplished even with just one arm, the experience of muscle relaxation will not be limited to just the one arm since all our extremities are tied to the same nervous system.

When we are active our muscles are quite naturally in a state of tension to accomplish whatever it is we are doing. When the neuromuscular system is in a relaxed state we have the feeling of heaviness in the extremities. It's quite common to be aware of this feeling just before going to sleep or upon waking up. In this first training we will focus on heaviness in the dominant arm.

Day One: Heaviness in the Dominant Arm

The phrase or formula we use for this training is *My right* (or *left,* if you are left-handed) *arm is heavy.* The arm starts at the shoulder and ends at the fingertips, so remember to concentrate on the whole arm during the training. It is important at this stage not to expect to feel anything happening. That is the key to passive volition. Don't expect that your arm will go heavy. The key to the training is to repeat the formulas and then passively observe what happens.

There are a few possibilities you might observe. Your arm might actually feel heavy. Some people describe the opposite—the arm feels lighter. Others, including myself, have found that during the very first session, before gaining the feeling of heaviness, which usually only occurs after many sessions, you feel pins and needles. For me this was not the debilitating feeling that occurs when an extremity "falls asleep" from being laid on or placed in an awkward position; rather, it was a tingly feeling in my fingers that was not unenjoyable. But no matter what happens on day one, we are on our way! I recommend that you repeat the dominant arm training several times during your first day. The more you can do it, the better. Don't forget to cancel between sets and at the end of each session.

+ Adopt a comfortable AT position and setting.
+ Engage in two minutes of passive breathing, slowly repeating *I breathe me.*
+ Take your mind to your dominant arm.
+ Repeat to yourself six times *My right* (or *left*) *arm is heavy.*
+ Turn your attention away from your dominant arm and say to yourself *I am very quiet.*
+ Remain relaxed for a minute or two.
+ Cancel (ending your session).
+ Repeat the whole sequence two more times to complete the session.

At this point I suggest you may wish to jot down your experiences in a notebook. I personally am not big on journaling, but for some people it is an effective tool. In my case it is amusing and enjoyable to go back years later and read what I wrote in my notebook about my first experiences with AT—both the amazing experiences and the frustrating ones.

Days Two to Four: Heaviness in Both Arms

Whether or not you experienced the feeling of heaviness, or anything else, on day one, it's good to keep on with the training. On days two to four we will include both arms in the training. Here is the procedure:

+ Adopt a comfortable AT position and setting.
+ Engage in passive breathing for two minutes, silently repeating *I breathe me.*
+ Passively focus on each arm, one at a time.
+ Starting with your dominant arm, silently repeat six times *My right* (or *left*) *arm is heavy.*
+ Go to your other arm and silently repeat six times *My left* (or *right*) *arm is heavy.*
+ Silently repeat three times *My arms are heavy.*
+ Turn your attention away from your arms and silently say *I am very quiet.*
+ Remain relaxed for a minute or two.
+ Cancel (cancel after each sequence, before repeating).
+ Repeat the whole sequence two more times to complete the session.

It is recommended that you do this training three times a day for days two through four.

Days Five through Seven: Heaviness in Both Arms and Legs

Adding both legs to the training is a big deal since our legs account for a major portion of muscles on our body. We're not going to focus on one leg at a time simply because by now you have already gone through enough sessions to be familiar with the process. When passively focusing on both arms and legs it is suggested that you try to feel all four extremities at the same time, including your torso, instead of moving your focus from side to side. This will provide a sense of unity and wholeness to the experience.

+ Adopt a comfortable AT position and setting.
+ For two minutes engage in passive breathing, silently repeating *I breathe me.*
+ Passively focus on each arm and each leg, one at a time.
+ Starting with your dominant arm, silently repeat six times *My right* (or *left*) *arm is heavy.*
+ Going to the other side, silently repeat six times *My left* (or *right*) *arm is heavy.*
+ Silently repeat three times *My arms are heavy.*
+ Silently repeat six times *My right* (or *left*) *leg is heavy.*
+ Silently repeat six times *My left* (or *right*) *leg is heavy.*
+ Silently repeat three times *My legs are heavy.*
+ Silently repeat three times *Both my arms and legs are heavy.*
+ Turn your attention away from your arms and legs and say to yourself *I am very quiet.*
+ Remain relaxed for a minute or two.
+ Cancel.
+ Repeat the sequence two more times to complete the session.

It is recommended that you repeat this training three times a day.

Congratulations on completing your first week of autogenic training! In the next training sessions we will add the training for your neck and back.

Training #3
Heaviness and Relaxation of the Neck and Back

Many of us carry a great deal of tension in the neck and back from various experiences in life, whether it be from work, relationships, repressed emotions, bad posture, etc. To get to a place where we can self-regulate the muscles where we typically hold these tensions is a great leap forward toward optimum health and well-being.

Unless you are a doctor or massage therapist it's not surprising that we don't realize how complex the muscles in our neck and back really are and therefore how susceptible they are to becoming tense and injured. A very brief overview will help us raise our awareness for our self-regulated training. Let's start with the neck. For our AT session we will be focusing on the back of the neck where these muscles attach to our back muscles.

The five major muscle groups in the back of the neck are the trapezius, the levator scapula, the splenius, the suboccipitals, and the posterior cervical muscles. The trapezius muscles connect between the neck, shoulders, and back; they are used when lifting the shoulder up toward the ears. The levator scapula connects the neck and the shoulder; it is used to lift the shoulders and turn the head. The splenius muscles connect the back of the head and neck with the vertebrae of the upper back; they are used to rotate the head and tilt it backward. The suboccipitals connect the skull with the top two vertebrae in the neck; they are used for the *yes* and *no* motions of your head, and for the side bending of the head. Lastly, the posterior cervical muscles along the back of the neck extend your head backward.

Now let's briefly look at the back muscles. The muscles of the back are divided into two specific groups: the extrinsic muscles, which are associated with upper extremity and shoulder movement, and the intrinsic muscles, which deal with movements of the vertebral column. Several small muscles in the cervical area of the vertebral column are also important. Intrinsic muscles, which stretch all the way from the pelvis to the cranium, help to maintain your posture and move the vertebral column. They're divided into three groups: the superficial layer, the intermediate layer, and the deep layer. The muscles in all of the layers are innervated by the posterior rami of spinal nerves. The superficial extrinsic muscles connect your upper extremities to the trunk, and they form the V-shaped musculature associated with the middle and upper back. They include the trapezius, latissimus dorsi, levator scapulae, and the rhomboids. Intermediate extrinsic muscles include the serratus posterior superior and inferior; most of their function is involved with respiration.

I've included this brief description of muscles simply to raise your awareness around the generic terms we use such as *neck* and *back*. During AT of the neck and back be aware of how many muscle groups you are actually passively connecting with. Our bodies are truly amazing!

Getting in touch with our neck and back muscles is a little more difficult than getting in touch with the arms and legs, which we are used to seeing as we use them. But with patience you will be able to do it. Since at this point you have a week of training behind you—around twenty-one sessions—it would be perfectly okay for someone to physically touch your muscles during the training if it's not too distracting, to bring your awareness to these areas. But this is certainly not necessary. For this training I have found that the rag-doll position (described in chapter 4) is the most effective, since the neck is not being supported. However, if you already have pain in your neck and this position makes it worse, please choose another position.

The phrase we use in this training is as simple as the others: *My neck and back are heavy*. The sequence of this training goes as follows:

+ Adopt a comfortable AT position and setting. The rag-doll position is recommended.
+ Engage in passive breathing for two minutes, silently repeating *I breathe me*.
+ Passively focus on each of the areas below one at a time.
+ Starting with your dominant arm, silently repeat three times *My right* (or *left*) *arm is heavy*.

+ Silently repeat three times *My arms and legs are heavy.*
+ Silently repeat six times *My neck and back are heavy.*
+ Turn your attention away from your neck and back and silently say *I am very quiet.*
+ Remain relaxed for a minute or two.
+ Cancel.
+ Repeat the sequence two more times to complete the session.

It is recommended that you do this training at least three times a day for a week.

Training #4

Vascular Dilation—The Experience of Warmth

Similar to how electrophysiological devices can measure muscular relaxation, AT heaviness trainings can also measure an observable change in warmth. Findings have shown a 6- to 8-degree increase in tissue warmth during the *My arms are warm* section of this training when a person is well trained. Training #4 affects the entire peripheral cardiovascular system—arteries, capillaries, and blood flow through muscles and skin. The procedure for the next week goes as follows:

Days One through Three

+ Engage in passive breathing for two minutes, slowly repeating *I breathe me.*
+ Passively focus on each of the areas below, one at a time.
+ Starting with your dominant arm, silently repeat three times *My right* (or *left*) *arm is heavy.*
+ Silently repeat three times *My arms and legs are heavy.*
+ Silently repeat six times *My right* (or *left*) *arm is warm.*
+ Silently repeat six times *My left* (or *right*) *arm is warm.*
+ Silently repeat six times *My arms are warm.*
+ Silently repeat three times *My neck and back are heavy.*
+ Turn your attention away from your neck and back and say to yourself *I am very quiet.*

+ Remain relaxed for a minute or two.
+ Cancel.
+ Repeat the whole sequence two more times to complete the session.

It is recommended that you do this training three times a day.

Days Four through Seven

+ Engage in passive breathing for two minutes, silently repeating *I breathe me.*
+ Passively focus on each of the areas below, one at a time.
+ Starting with your dominant arm, silently repeat three times *My right* (or *left*) arm is heavy.
+ Silently repeat three times *My arms and legs are heavy.*
+ Silently repeat three times *My right* (or *left*) arm is warm.
+ Silently repeat three times *My left* (or *right*) arm is warm.
+ Silently repeat three times *My arms are warm.*
+ Silently repeat three times *My right* (or *left*) leg is warm.
+ Silently repeat three times *My left* (or *right*) leg is warm.
+ Silently repeat three times *My legs are warm.*
+ Silently repeat six times *My arms and legs are warm.*
+ Silently repeat three times *My neck and back are heavy.*
+ Turn your attention away from your neck and back and silently say *I am very quiet.*
+ Remain relaxed for a minute or two.
+ Cancel.
+ Repeat the sequence two more times to complete the session.

It is recommended that you do this training three times a day. Don't forget to take notes if you've been keeping them.

Training #5
Regulation of the Heart

The expressions *a broken heart, to have a big heart, to follow your heart, from the heart, a heart of gold,* etc. don't have anything to do with the biological functioning of the heart, yet these metaphors clearly demonstrate the important emotional function of this vital organ. So at this point in the training let's take a few moments to discuss the emotional aspects of the training.

During this AT training you have been intentionally making time for yourself in an undisturbed, quiet place, and by this time you've been doing this for a few weeks. Having established this routine is quite a significant achievement, and already it has no doubt led to your experiencing increased vitality, better concentration, and higher self-awareness. However, this increased self-awareness can also bring up feelings that need attention.

When suppressed feelings and emotions come up during AT we can easily lose our passive concentration. This is not all bad. In many cases it is a sign that you should slow down with the training and clear up unresolved issues, which will ultimately only help you in life. For those of you who find yourselves in this situation, bringing these issues to light through AT and then dealing with them may in the long run be even more important than the AT training itself. The training we are doing, making time for ourselves and discovering the functioning of our body, will necessarily lead to altered brain activity and states of consciousness. This is exactly the self-generated training we are seeking.

At this point in the training (sometimes earlier) clients often ask me why they should cancel between sets, stating that they were just getting into it but then had to cancel. The reason for this is that we need to have a place to finish and then start again; otherwise we may forget the procedure as we get lost in it. At the end of your quiet time it's better to cancel and then start the next set. Keep in mind that the cancel can be performed very gently, peacefully, and gracefully. You are simply outstretching your arms and hands from the prayer position and gently inhaling and exhaling. This is the recommended way to end a set and prepare for the next one. Moreover, by canceling we bring much more self-awareness into the ritual, as canceling helps to frame the experience.

Thus opening a set with passive breathing, and ending by canceling, are the two bookends of the experience.

Now let's get back to the training. The phrase we use in this part of the training is *My heartbeat is calm and strong.* When we say the phrase to ourselves we take our mind to the area of our body where our heart is. Your heart is about the size of your fist and is located behind and to the left of your sternum. During the training we can also pay passive attention to any place in our body where we feel a pulse. This could be a hand, a foot, or your temple, neck, or any other place where you feel a pulse. For example, I have had multiple injuries to muscles around my left rib cage so I often feel my pulse there during AT.

Thus far during AT training we have learned the experience of generating warmth by passively connecting with our peripheral cardiovascular system and experiencing vascular dilation. We've experienced muscular relaxation through passively concentrating on heaviness and our breath. The next step is to combine the heaviness and warmth experiences, adding the heart. The formula for this week is as follows:

+ Adopt a comfortable AT position and setting.
+ Engage in passive breathing for two minutes, silently repeating *I breathe me.*
+ Passively focus on each of the areas below, one at a time.
+ Starting with your dominant arm, silently repeat three times *My right* (or *left*) *arm is heavy.*
+ Silently repeat six times *My arms and legs are heavy.*
+ Concentrate on your heartbeat and silently repeat six times *My heartbeat is calm and strong.*
+ While still aware of your heartbeat say to yourself *I am very quiet.*
+ Remain relaxed for a minute or two.
+ Cancel.
+ Repeat the whole sequence two more times to complete the session.

I recommend that you do this session three times a day.

Training #6
Solar Plexus—Warmth in the Abdomen

The celiac plexus, also known as the solar plexus because of its radiating nerve fibers, is a complex network of nerves (a.k.a. a plexus) located in the abdomen, where the celiac trunk, superior mesenteric artery, and renal arteries branch from the abdominal aorta. It is in back of the stomach and the omental bursa, and in front of the crura of the diaphragm, on the level of the first lumbar vertebra. Or in layman's terms: if you look down to your belly and put a finger halfway between your naval and the lower end of your sternum where your rib cage comes together just below your chest, that's the center of the solar plexus.

The solar plexus is the center of the autonomic nervous system. It is such a vital nerve center that some martial artists and boxers target this area because trauma there can literally strike at the heart of an opponent, paralyzing the heart and other vital organs. But our aim is obviously the opposite. As a key nervous center of the body we want to try to connect with it.

Except for the next (and last) training in this section having to do with the head, the solar plexus is the most difficult to connect with and may take more time than the previous trainings. This is mainly due to the fact that unlike the arms or legs, we never actually see this plexus, and we never feel it either, unlike our breath or heartbeat. But with patience and practice it is possible to passively focus on this very important area. In AT training we want to connect with this area because through the many interconnected nerves there such as the vagus nerve (which interfaces with parasympathetic control of the heart and digestive tract), the solar plexus serves as a relay station directly from the organs to the brain. Through hormones and numerous chemicals it also relays information about the extremely important immune system. So in a nutshell, the solar plexus gives the brain the information it needs to regulate the functioning of the body; by getting in touch with it through AT we can passively affect brain function. In all the previous trainings we have indirectly affected the solar plexus through our passive actions. Now we will go to the center with the intention of further promoting self-regulation and self-healing.

As I have already said, this solar plexus training is not easy, so it is important to persevere. At this point I usually tell my clients that it's perfectly fine not to slavishly stick to my instructions. Yes, I have many years of experience, but we are all different, and you may have gone even deeper in your other practices than I have. So basically what I'm saying here is that these formulas work for a reason; they're time-tested. You can't go wrong by using them. But they are also not carved in stone. If you don't say a phrase exactly three or more times, no big deal. At this point in your training you can move as fluidly as your internal awareness decides.

Although you have probably felt this already during your AT training, the solar plexus training can bring about deep states of altered consciousness if and when you connect to this central point of the nervous system. During this part of the training it is common for clients to report feelings of weightlessness and floating, and even out-of-body experiences where they see themselves from outside their body, usually from above. I have never heard anyone say these experiences were negative; to the contrary, they always seem to be very inspiring and somehow enlightening to people. In a few of the practices in the primal mind part of this book we will intentionally seek these kinds of experiences. However, if you get into one of these experiences and feel too uncomfortable, then simply cancel out immediately.

The formula for the coming week is as follows:

+ Adopt a comfortable AT position and setting.
+ Engage in passive breathing for two minutes, silently repeating *I breathe me.*
+ Passively focus on each of the areas below, one at a time.
+ Starting with your dominant arm, silently repeat three times *My right* (or *left*) *arm is heavy.*
+ Silently repeat three times *My arms and legs are heavy and warm.*
+ Silently repeat three times *My heartbeat is calm and strong.*

✦ Silently repeat six times *My solar plexus is warm.*

✦ While still aware of the area of your solar plexus, say to yourself *I am very quiet.*

✦ Remain relaxed for a minute or two.

✦ Cancel.

✦ Repeat the whole sequence three times to complete the session.

I recommend this exercise be done three times daily.

At this stage it's perfectly fine to linger in one area if that intuitively feels right; however, I advise against changing the order of the sequence because this order stimulates muscles and nerves in a progression that builds momentum. If you have not been taking notes about what is happening during your training sessions, these sessions are perfect for noting sensations, feelings, and any experiences or no experiences. Even if you don't experience or feel anything unusual, the health benefits of the deep states of relaxation of AT are well worth the effort.

Training #7
Cooling the Forehead

The brain has four distinct regions termed *lobes:* the frontal lobe, the temporal lobe, the parietal lobe, and the occipital lobe. The frontal lobe is the largest region of our brain, sitting just behind the forehead. It is a highly complex, specialized region that helps to control many different and important functions: organization, concept formation, mental flexibility, personality, execution of behavior (the frontal lobe is often referred to as the *executive system*), abstract reasoning, problem solving, planning, judgment, ethical behavior, inhibition, expressive language, and attention.

Passively getting in touch with this part of the brain through AT has many benefits in terms of relaxation, peace, and well-being. However, this particular training is by far the most challenging to accomplish yet. To give you an idea: AT students and teachers report that all the previous trainings have anywhere from an 80 to 90 percent success rate for the goals of the trainings.* But the forehead-cooling training results show somewhere in the vicinity of a 40 percent success rate. For those who report feeling the cooling, it usually takes anywhere from seven to fourteen days to learn. The feeling is not exactly cold, but rather closer to the feeling you experience when you blow on the back of your hand. But it doesn't really matter if you don't feel your forehead cooling; regardless of your experience, it doesn't take anything away from the relaxation, peace, body connection, and health benefits that practicing any part of AT produces.

The cooling of the forehead training can be likened to the relaxing effect of a cool (not cold) cloth on the forehead. I recommend doing this training three times a day. The sequence goes as follows:

+ Adopt a comfortable AT position and setting.
+ Engage in passive breathing for two minutes, silently repeating *I breathe me.*
+ Passively focus on each of the areas below, one at a time.
+ Starting with your dominant arm, silently repeat three times *My right* (or *left*) *arm is heavy.*
+ Silently repeat three times *My arms and legs are heavy and warm.*
+ Silently repeat three times *My heartbeat is calm and strong.*
+ Silently repeat three times *My solar plexus is warm.*
+ Silently repeat six times *My forehead is pleasantly cool.*
+ Silently repeat three times *My neck and back are warm.*
+ While still aware of the areas of your neck and back, say to yourself *I am very quiet.*
+ Remain relaxed for a minute or two.
+ Cancel.
+ Repeat the sequence two more times to complete the session.

ᘓ

You've now completed the seven standard autogenic training formulas. But there is much more to come. There are two things to remember

---

*Whether this is optimistic or not, I don't know. But these figures seem accurate for my students. Almost anyone can master AT if they take the time and have the desire.

now: It usually takes anywhere from four to six months to master these techniques, so keep practicing. And as previously mentioned, these trainings can be practiced anywhere (refer to chapter 4 for suggestions). Once you have mastered the first seven trainings you can use them whenever you feel necessary, especially when combined with the following trainings. At this point it is not necessary to train three times a day anymore, and you can use a singular training or any combination of the trainings at any time. Train at your discretion, but keep training!

Glean the benefits of the trainings you have mastered but continue to practice them, and keep trying to master the ones you haven't. Warmth in the solar plexus (training #6) and cooling the forehead (training #7) can be elusive experiences. If you are initially stumped by them simply pick any of the other trainings you have mastered and do them properly first, then try trainings 6 and 7 again in the same session. If you haven't yet mastered all seven of the standard trainings it is fine to continue on with the trainings to come. Many times as we learn the upcoming trainings it is easier to come back and master trainings 6 and 7.

6

AUTOGENIC TRAINING WITH POSITIVE AFFIRMATIONS

I hope the seven standard AT formulas have proven valuable to you and that you continue with your practice. However, AT is certainly not limited to physiological concerns. In this chapter we will use our experience with the deep states of passive volition and focus that we have learned and developed through the seven exercises and apply them to affirm the positive aspects of our being in order to deal with those aspects of ourselves that we want to change or modify. By doing so, we open ourselves to unlimited personal growth and optimum health.

Injecting affirmations into our AT formulas is a powerful way to enhance our lives or make needed changes. Affirmations are positive statements or "self-scripts" that can condition the subconscious mind, especially in a deep state of relaxation such as that induced by AT. Affirmations help you develop a more positive perception of yourself and can help you change negative, self-sabotaging behaviors. They can help undo the damage caused by old negative programming, those scripts we picked up a long time ago that contribute to a negative self-perception. Affirmations are easy to create and use, and I am going to provide some examples in this chapter, but you will need dedication to make them work.

Note that you have to be careful to be realistic about what you try to work on. For example, if you want to lose weight, injecting the statement

I will lose weight into your formula will not make you lose weight without a corresponding weight-loss plan. If you are on a proven plan for losing weight, the affirmation will provide more force and plant a seed of confidence within you. The same with completing any other kind of project—a firm plan to accomplish the task is necessary, while the affirmation can help you carry the momentum to actually achieve the goal.

Here are some suggestions pertaining to affirmations:

- Think about your positive attributes. We rarely focus on those things we really like about ourselves, and instead we often choose to dwell on things we'd like to change. Taking an inventory will help you break that cycle, and using affirmations as an aid to help you appreciate who you truly are will give you the confidence you need to become who you want to be. Take stock of yourself by making an inventory of your best qualities, abilities, or other attributes. Are you a hard worker? Are you sensitive to other people's feelings? Write each quality down in a short sentence, starting with "I" and using the present tense: "I am confident," for example, or "I am generous."

- Think about which negative scripts you want to counteract, or what positive goals you want to accomplish. Affirmations can be extremely useful in counteracting the negative perceptions you have developed about your appearance, your abilities, or your potential. Affirmations can also help you achieve specific goals, such as losing weight or quitting smoking. Make a list of your goals or the harmful self-perceptions you want to change.

- Prioritize your list of things to work on. You may find that you have a lot of goals or that you need to work on many negative scripts. It's best, however, to concentrate on just a few affirmations at a time, so choose those that are most important or most urgent and work with them first. Once you see improvement in those areas or you accomplish those goals, you can develop new affirmations for other items on your list. You can try using as many affirmations as you want at any given time, but you may want to start by using no more than five.

- Write down the affirmations you will use to influence future changes. Be short, clear, and positive.

- There are two kinds of future-oriented affirmations you can use to work toward goals. With "I can" statements, you write down a statement affirming the fact that you can achieve your goal(s). For example, if you want to quit smoking, a statement such as, "I can quit smoking" is typical. But many experts recommend that you avoid any sort of negative connotation, so that you would instead say something like, "I can free myself from smoking," or "I can become smoke-free."

- With "I will" statements, you write down a statement affirming that today you will actually use your ability to achieve a desired goal. So following the above example, you could say, "I will be smoke-free today," or "I will smoke fewer cigarettes today than yesterday." Again, the affirmation should use positive language and should simply express what you will do today to achieve the longer-term goal.

- Match up some of your positive attributes with your goals. Which of your positive qualities that you have affirmed will help you achieve the goals you have set? If you're overcoming the desire to smoke, for example, you may need willpower or courage, or you may need to reflect on the fact that you are a smart person or that you care about your family. Select two or three of these affirmations to support your goal-oriented affirmations, and say those in addition to your specific goal-oriented statements.

When coming up with goal-setting affirmations, make sure they are simple, concise, and objective oriented. For example, "I will finish my master's degree this semester on schedule," or "I will abstain from yelling at my children." Only you can formulate your plans and goals. Below are some examples of non-goal-oriented affirmations that in general can add greatly to your consciousness and subconscious when combined with AT:

I love and approve of myself.
I adopt the mind-set to praise myself.
I see the perfection in all my flaws and in my genius.
I fully approve of who I am, even as I get better.
I press on because I believe in my path.
The past has no power over me anymore.
I take pleasure in my own solitude.
I am confident that I can overcome my disease (or disability).
I am deeply fulfilled with who I am now.
My body is healthy and functioning in a very good way.
My mind is calm.
My thoughts are under control.
I radiate love and happiness.

Since you are already familiar with the standard formulas as outlined in the previous chapter, you can create your own for your goal-oriented and positive affirmations by using the standard formulas as a template. Whatever you decide to do, I suggest you always begin with passive breathing and heaviness in your dominant arm, because this sets the stage for passive volition, quiets the mind, and relaxes the body. There are two recommended formulas I share with my clients, and both are listed below. The first one interjects the affirmation between each standard formula, and the second places the affirmation between the forehead and neck/back formula. This example could be for someone who lacks confidence or who is very shy:

Training #8
Adding Affirmations Formulas

+ Adopt a comfortable AT position and setting.
+ Engage in passive breathing for two minutes, silently repeating *I breathe me.*

+ Passively focus on each of the areas below, one at a time.
+ Starting with your dominant arm, silently repeat three times *My right* (or *left*) *arm is heavy.*
+ Silently repeat six times *I can be assertive.*
+ Silently repeat three times *My arms and legs are warm.*
+ Silently repeat six times *I can be assertive.*
+ Silently repeat three times *My heartbeat is calm and strong.*
+ Silently repeat six times *I can be assertive.*
+ Silently repeat three times *My neck and back are warm.*
+ While still aware of the areas of your neck and back, say to yourself *I am very quiet.*
+ Remain relaxed for a minute or two.
+ Cancel.
+ Repeat this sequence two more times.

You have seven different standard formulas to choose from; you could use any of them or just the ones that you feel you have mastered. Some people prefer warmth to heaviness, or solar plexus rather than neck and back. Some go the traditional route and do all seven formulas and inject their own formula(s), which is a great idea. It's up to you.

Another example of how to inject an affirmation is as follows:

+ Adopt a comfortable AT position and setting.
+ Engage in passive breathing for two minutes, silently repeating *I breathe me.*
+ Passively focus on each of the areas below, one at a time.
+ Starting with your dominant arm, silently repeat three times *My right* (or *left*) *arm is heavy.*
+ Silently repeat three times *My arms and legs are heavy and warm.*
+ Silently repeat three times *My solar plexus is warm.*
+ Silently repeat six times *I can be assertive.*
+ Silently repeat three times *My heartbeat is calm and strong.*
+ While still aware of your heartbeat say to yourself *I am very quiet.*
+ Remain relaxed for a minute or two.

✦ Cancel.

✦ Repeat the sequence two more times.

My last suggestion—and this is an important one: always perform a standard formula without an affirmation as the final sequence. The standard formulas are tangible physiological processes that ground your being.

7

AUTOGENIC TRAINING AND MEDICAL/ PSYCHOSOMATIC/ PSYCHIATRIC DISORDERS

In Japan and parts of Europe AT is a very popular adjunct to traditional medical practices and therapies. Wolfgang Linden, a psychologist who teaches at the University of British Columbia whose clinical specialties include health psychology, psychophysiology, cardiac rehabilitation, hypertension, and psychological adjustment to cancer, says, "The available literature on AT is vast and suggests that AT has been effectively used for literally any medical/psychosomatic/psychiatric disorder that may possess a psychological component."[1]

AT's range of psychotherapeutic applications is extensive and includes multiple sclerosis, tremors, tics, facial spasms, neuralgia, phantom limb syndrome, narcolepsy, brain injury, epilepsy, cerebral palsy, manic depression, schizophrenia, paranoia, anxiety, dissociative disorder, phobias, obsessive-compulsive disorder, hypochondriasis, sexual deviation, addiction (smoking, alcoholism, drugs, etc.), obsessive masturbation, somnambulism, writer's block, stuttering, and sleep disorders. It is highly effective for those seeking improved performance in sports, industry, and education.

Medical applications of AT include disorders of deglutition (swallowing), dyspepsia, peptic ulcer, biliary disorders, ulcerative colitis, irritable colon, constipation, food allergies, obesity, anorexia nervosa, sinus bradycardia, tachycardia, arrhythmia, extrasystoles (premature cardiac contraction), left mammary pain, angina pectoris, myocardial infarction, cardiac neurosis (anxiety concerning the state of the heart), high blood pressure, Raynaud's disease, hemorrhoids, blushing (endothoracic sympathectomy), tension and migraine headaches, bronchial asthma, pulmonary tuberculosis, diabetes mellitus, thyroid dysfunctions, lipid metabolism disorders, tetany (muscle cramps), arthritis, nonarticular rheumatism, low-back pain, hemophilia, sexual dysfunctions, gynecologic disorders, pregnancy complications and labor pain, skin disorders, dental pain, and preparation for surgery.

As we can see, AT can be employed for a wide variety of conditions; most in the medical category are best administered by health-care professionals, with AT serving as an adjunct therapy. But as we know, we can also use AT for our personal situations. I have used AT successfully for the chronic pain in my rotator cuff from rock climbing and for pain as a result of cutting my knee with a chain saw, to give just a couple of examples.

Here are a few examples of affirmations to address different conditions:

Sleep Disorders
I know I'll sleep through the night.
Darkness makes me comfortable and sleepy.
Warmth and comfort make me sleepy.

Angina (Chest Pain)
My heartbeat is calm.
My chest is loose and warm.

Asthma
My breathing is comfortable and calm.
My lungs are open and free.
My throat is warm (or cool).

Obesity

I know I can stick to my diet.
Small meals are adequate for me.
I don't get hungry between meals.

Pain

I am unaffected by my pain.
I can free myself from any pain.
As I relax, the pain drains out of my body.

Sexual Problems

My erection is strong and well maintained.
My ejaculation is easily delayed.
I know I can satisfy my partner.

Smoking

Smoking revolts me.
Tobacco tastes foul and revolting.
Smoking is not for me.

Here's a sample session that adds a healing affirmation, which I used for a knee injury:

Training #9
Adding Healing Formulas

✦ Adopt a comfortable AT position and setting.

✦ Engage in passive breathing for two minutes, silently repeating *I breathe me.*

✦ Passively focus on each of the areas below, one at a time.

✦ Starting with your dominant arm, silently repeat three times *My right* (or *left*) *arm is heavy.*

✦ Silently repeat six times *The pain in my knee is diminishing.*

✦ Silently repeat three times *My heartbeat is calm and strong.*

+ Silently repeat six times *The pain in my knee is diminishing.*
+ Silently repeat three times *My arms and legs are warm.*
+ Silently repeat six times *The pain in my knee is diminishing.*
+ Silently repeat three times *My neck and back are warm.*
+ While still aware of the areas of your neck and back say to yourself *I am very quiet.*
+ Remain relaxed for a minute or two.
+ Cancel.
+ Repeat this sequence two more times.

The above exercise greatly helped me manage the pain I had as a result of an accident in which I cut my knee with a chain saw. I used this formula at least three times a day and sometimes more frequently throughout the healing process, especially when I was in excruciating pain (I had to crawl to the bathroom). I have had many clients who came up with their own personal variations on the standard formulas to successfully help with everything from the common cold to more serious problems like irritable bowel syndrome. For me the proof for anything lies in the results. The fact is, AT can be employed successfully as a powerful mode of self-healing.

PART THREE

Advanced Autogenic Training Techniques

8
VISUALIZATION AND AUTOGENIC TRAINING

Dr. Johannes Schultz, the originator of AT, together with his protégé Dr. Wolfgang Luthe (1922–1985), also a medical doctor who, among other appointments, served as professor of psychophysiologic therapy at the International Institute of Stress, in Montreal, Canada, developed seven visualization trainings (sometimes referred to as *meditations*) designed to be used as extensions of the seven standard AT formulas. These upper-level, advanced, or second-stage trainings are found in very few English translations of the work of Schultz and Luthe. Nevertheless, by now we have gathered sufficient information about these advanced trainings such that when combined with my many years of experience working with AT in group settings and with individuals, I can now offer this information in this book.

Similar to the seven standard trainings, the seven visualization trainings in this chapter each have their own themes and goals. However, once you are *inside* the visualization trainings you will find that they are much more free-form than the basic seven trainings. For this reason, the prerequisite for these advanced trainings is mastery of the seven standard formulas. One should be able to promptly enter an autogenic state within one to two minutes before beginning any of these advanced trainings. I have found that in the latter part of training in the seven standard formulas, many people (myself included) begin to see in their mind's eye the spontaneous manifestation of colors. The evocation of colors is an upper-level AT training, so if you are already seeing colors during your standard AT sessions it's a sign that you are ready for the advanced visualization trainings presented here.

During my early research on advanced AT it became clear that the various translations of Schultz and Luthe had resulted in variations on the seven visualization exercises. It may also have been that early on the therapists using these techniques adapted them for their own specific uses. In any case, these variations aren't too different to be radically important. I've tried all three of the series examples in table 8.1 (page 68) in my workshops, and in doing so the participants and I have come up with our own series (the "suggested series" in table 8.1), which I think takes the most effective steps from all three. One thing I have found in most of the translations of the advanced trainings is that Schultz and Luthe encouraged combining the series *after mastering them separately.* First, master the series separately, then feel free to combine them if that's the way your session flows.

With this in mind, feel free to try all four examples in table 8.1 (page 68) or come up with your own after you have successfully experienced the various formulas. The "suggested series" of steps below has proven to be the most effective in my work.

To begin this advanced training we'll start with a meditative technique described by Shultz and Luthe as "voluntary rotation of the eyeballs upward and inward, looking at the center of the forehead."[1] Notably a great many paintings and statues of both Eastern and Western mystics depict figures with their eyes in just this position. That's because many forms of meditation employ this technique, as it has been proven to induce and increase alpha rhythms in the brain. Alpha rhythms are patterns of smooth, electrical oscillations in the brain that reflect a transcendent, dynamic state of being. Since 1935, scientists and researchers of meditation have proven that masters of such practices as hatha yoga, Zen, and Transcendental Meditation can alter their alpha brain rhythms, heart rate, and skin conductance. Research on this continues, and we will delve into this more in chapter 9, on autogenic meditation. For now let's look at what happens during an alpha state.

TABLE 8.1. EXAMPLES OF ADVANCED AT VISUALIZATION SERIES

	Step 1	Step 2	Step 3	Step 4	Step 5	Step 6	Step 7
Series 1	Spontaneous evocation of colors	Evocation of colors on demand	Visualizing objects	Visualizing a person	Imaginative evocation of concepts	Using self-directed questions	
Series 2	Controlling the evocation of colors	Visualization of concrete objects	Imagery of abstract concepts	Mental image of a person	Visualization of a bridge	Visualization or walking or running	Visualization of a door
Series 3	Basic meditation posture and eye position	Visualization of vivid basic colors	Visualization of static objects	Visualization of abstract concepts	Increased participation—"filmstrips" and "multichromatic Cinerama"	Visualization of other persons	
Suggested Series	Spontaneous evocation of colors	Evocation of colors on demand	Visualizing objects	Visualization of people	Visualization of abstract concepts	Increased participation—"filmstrips"	Using self-directed questions

Without having an EEG to measure brain waves or an instrument that measures galvanic skin response (the alteration in the electrical resistance of the skin associated with sympathetic nerve discharge), we can simply see and subjectively feel the characteristics of alpha waves, which include the following:

- Breathing and heart rate slow down.
- Subject becomes completely passive, both mentally and physically.
- Body temperature may rise, sometimes to the point of perspiring.
- Subject may see colors with eyes closed.
- Eyes may automatically move rapidly (called *rapid eye movement,* or REM), which one also experiences when dreaming.
- Galvanic skin response goes up.
- The body may sway slowly and pleasantly as energy is released and consciousness expands.

Visualization has historically been a key practice in most if not all Eastern mystical traditions, and more recently it has been adopted by many people in the West because of its effectiveness in dealing with a variety of situations and conditions. Over the centuries, thousands of volumes have been written attesting to the esoteric and psychological processes involved in visualization. In autogenic visualization, we intentionally cultivate an alert, focused awareness while at the same time detaching from thoughts and emotions. This process does not drain our energy like most circumstances in life. Quite the contrary, most people who practice autogenic visualization and autogenic meditation report having much more available energy than they otherwise would have. And when we focus our visualizations on the above list of suggested training steps (table 8.1), we can gain profound insights about life.

Throughout this discussion about AT I have emphasized passive volition as being key. During the visualization trainings this is especially true. Visualization is employed in other esoteric and meditative modalities in many ways. Sometimes visualization techniques begin the process, and other times they are used to deepen an altered state of consciousness or to channel energy toward a specific goal or purpose. The seemingly contrary nature of passive volition, in which we are essentially doing without doing, is just as true for the visualization trainings as it is for the standard AT formulas. With our standard AT formulas we plant the seed and simply let it grow. For example, if I try really hard to feel my dominant arm get heavy, it won't. Neither will I feel warmth in my solar plexus if I concentrate with all my might on this result. The same is true for autogenic visualization techniques: we plant the seed and simply let it take hold and grow. It's true that autogenic visualization is much more dynamic than the standard formulas, and you have more of an ability to control what you visualize. But the more passively you can accomplish your visualizations, the more successful the outcome.

Now let's go back to the suggested position of the eyeballs to begin the training. I'm not counting this step as a visualization because it is basically a preparatory step. However, similar to *I breathe me* in standard AT, it is an extremely important and powerful first step in the visualization process. The act of "voluntary rotation of the eyeballs upward and inward, looking at the center of the forehead," as described by Schultz and Luthe, is exactly the same as the yogic practice of focusing on the Ajna, or third-eye chakra (although Schultz and Luthe made no mention of the third eye in their writings). In yogic traditions the chakras, of which there are seven major ones, are basically the energetic centers of our ethereal body. We will discuss this more in the next chapter.

In any case, the act of beginning the visualization training with this movement of the eyes is very effective. For some people this is an easy thing to do and they get it right away, no problem. For others (like me) it takes a little practice. Here are the instructions for opening the third eye, followed by some helpful hints:

Preparing for Visualization—Opening the Third Eye

✦ Adopt an AT body position or if you practice yoga you can get into a half-lotus or similar seated posture.

+ Close your eyes.
+ Relax and breathe normally for a few moments until you feel still and quiet.
+ Now concentrate on the middle of your forehead for a few moments while keeping your eyes straight ahead under your closed lids.
+ After a few moments of concentrating your attention on the center of your forehead, move your eyes upward and inward (or inward and upward) so that they are directed to the area about two centimeters above the space right between your eyebrows.

That's it. This is actually very simple to do but sometimes not so easy for some of us. The first time I tried it I tried too hard and my chin went up so high that the bottom back of my head practically touched my back while my eyes were straining so hard they hurt. These first attempts were the complete opposite of what we are trying to do here, so on to the helpful hints:

• It is vitally important that you remain completely relaxed. Your facial muscles in particular should be in a state of complete repose.
• If you are in a seated position it is perfectly normal that you raise your chin slightly—that's actually how the yogis do it. But the key word is *slightly*—one inch above the horizontal plane is the most you want. However, I suggest starting with the chin in a comfortable horizontal position and then make minor adjustments as your intuition dictates.
• When adjusting the eyes, first move them gently toward the center and then slightly upward so that you are looking just slightly above—about 20 degrees—the center of your eyebrows. If you look too far up for any length of time your eyes will become strained. This position of the eyes should be completely comfortable.
• I learned this from a respected yogi: while breathing normally, tilt head down until your chin touches the chest. As you tilt your head down look up as much as you can without straining your eyes. Then lift your chin back up to the horizontal position while

letting your eyes lift to just above your eyebrows, and at the same time bring them inward.

- It is normal for people to see flickering lights or have twitching eyelids or facial muscles around the eyes in the beginning. This is what I experienced. This is normal and will dissipate with practice, but just be sure this is not occurring because you are straining or trying too hard. (This can also happen if you recently drank coffee or some other caffeinated beverage that has gotten you wired.) All you need to do is remain relaxed and practice.

For simplicity in the text that follows I will refer to this preliminary eye position as *the third eye*.

Training #10
Spontaneous Evocation of Colors

Once you feel comfortable adopting and holding the third-eye position, it's time for the first training in the advanced series, which has to do with visualizing colors.

Begin by completing a good session of any of the standard formulas you have mastered, but don't cancel at the end. During the standard AT session you may see colors or lights as if projected on your closed eyelids like a movie screen. This is quite common for people who are in the later stages of learning the standard formulas and for those for who have mastered them. If you are not already seeing colors simply remain relaxed; they may appear in five minutes or half an hour. Just be patient, be passive, and have a good standard AT session. Spontaneous colors and lights come in many forms, and in this first training simply passively watch them and don't try to control them. I have seen lots of different color schemes and patterns. The most common ones reported by my clients are static dots of different or single colors, slowly moving dots, colored dots moving together in a formation, swirls of multiple or single colors, and random diluted colors that are hazy or smoky. It may be that you see none of this and instead see your own color patterns.

At some point you will probably note a merging of what you see into a single color. We call this your *base color,* which simply means that during your regular AT session or when you are very relaxed you most commonly see this particular color. Remember, being able to perceive colors and color patterns could take days' or weeks' worth of practice, but once you get the hang of it your base color will appear very rapidly, sometimes even unexpectedly during your regular AT session.

✦ Perform a good standard AT session, but don't cancel at the end.
✦ Now concentrate on the middle of your forehead for a few moments, then gently move your eyes inward, then upward, toward the third eye.
✦ Maintain your passive AT state for twenty to thirty minutes or until colors begin.
✦ Passively observe whatever colors and color patterns arise for ten to fifteen minutes.
✦ Cancel.

Training #11
Evocation of Colors on Demand

Now it's time to use passive volition to evoke your base color and other colors. Some colors like yellow, orange, and certain shades of purple usually produce a feeling of warmth. With red be careful. If you see red and are still comfortably relaxed, then fine. If you start to feel agitated or aggressive, cancel immediately. Blue and green are known to have a cooling effect similar to training #7, cooling the forehead (chapter 5).

From here it is perfectly natural and advisable to visualize colors in formations such as hazes, clouds, or something that resembles colored shadows slowly moving across your visual field. In time you can visualize geometric patterns, which often morph into a kaleidoscope of colors, shapes, fractals, patterns, spirals, checkerboards, grids, webs, and funnels either static or moving. If what you are seeing is static, then try experimenting with movement, such as making your vision bigger or smaller, turning, curving, or rotating. Some researchers claim that visions similar to the ones described here happen spontaneously while we are awake and when we are sleeping, although we do not consciously acknowledge them due to our normally active psychological functioning. It is only through passive volition that we can consciously tune in to these visions.

+ Perform a good standard AT session, but don't cancel at the end.
+ Now concentrate on the middle of your forehead for a few moments, then gently move your eyes inward, then upward toward the third eye.
+ Maintain your passive AT state for twenty to thirty minutes, or until colors begin to form.
+ Bring to mind specific colors and observe how they manifest. Visualize colors taking shape and moving.
+ Cancel.

Though there is no set time limit for doing this, I have found that for most people forty-five minutes to an hour is an average length of time for the entire session.

Training #12
Visualization of Objects

The third training in this series involves visualizing and holding an image of a particular object. This can be anything that spontaneously comes to mind or an image that you plan ahead of time. Some people like to visualize special personal items or an object that evokes pleasant memories or peaceful feelings. Common objects to use in this visualization are vases, flowers, fruit (apples are a common motif when working with an AT instructor). In my first attempt at this I spontaneously envisioned a garden rake, of all things, probably because I had been using one in my yard the previous two days.

In this training we are not going for movement. A static image is fine. Try to visualize a few different items with each session. It is helpful to visualize objects on a dark background. Even though you are exploring the visualization of objects, sometimes you might see your base color instead. That's perfectly fine; simply attempt to passively visualize your object with your color as the background.

This training has been found to be much more difficult than the color trainings. It's not easy to passively conjure up an image of an object in your mind's eye. Oftentimes when we are successful, the image stays only fleetingly; other times the image may be hazy, unclear, or blurry. Patience and practice are key here. Objects will gradually become clearer with practice.

Sometimes when people have difficulties with this visualization I suggest a complementary technique to try. This involves choosing something that you are not emotionally attached to and holding it in your hands. I like to use fruit because we can add smell to the equation. So let's say you choose a lemon. Hold the lemon in your hands and concentrate on it. Focus on how it feels, think about how it tastes, smell it, look intently at its bright color. Now close your eyes and still see the lemon. Do this three times or more until you can still see the lemon when you close your eyes. This can help open up your inner vision. Once you can do this sit in a room and randomly pick out an object that you don't hold in your hands. For example, I can see a portable fan from where I am sitting as I write this. I can focus on it for a few seconds, close my eyes, and still see it. I don't see it as clearly as with my eyes open, but it is still there in my mind's eye.

Once you are able to visualize objects, whether with complete clarity or not, I recommend that you alter the cancel step somewhat. I train people to cancel between each object, but in a different way from the standard cancellation. Here it is best to back off the image first, with statements such as:

> The (name of object) *has become less clear.*
> The (name of object) *is gradually receding.*
> The (name of object) *has completely disappeared.*

Then briefly focus on your body with statements such as:

My breathing is normal, my heartbeat is calm and strong.
My body feels relaxed and peaceful.
I open my eyes in a state of tranquillity but fully alert.

You can use these statements to cancel gradually, or find your own verbiage—whatever works best for you. Do this for each object.

The following is a sample exercise for visualizing objects:

+ If you are going to choose a specific object do it now and concentrate on it for a few moments. Sometimes naming it out loud and describing it out loud helps to visualize it later.
+ Perform a good standard AT session, but don't cancel at the end.
+ Now concentrate on the middle of your forehead for a few moments, then gently move your eyes inward, then upward toward your third eye.
+ Maintain your passive AT state for twenty to thirty minutes and begin to visualize your first object.
+ Visualize a few more objects in succession, canceling gradually as described above between each object and at the end of your session.

Remember, this training may take longer than the others because it is an advanced technique.

Training #13
Visualization of People

This training is similar to the previous one but now instead of an object you visualize a person. At first it's best to visualize neutral people—people whom you know reasonably well but are not emotionally attached to. Once you have accomplished that part of the exercise you can gradually move on to other, more significant people in your life. It is common, especially in the beginning, for images of people to seem hazy and fade rather quickly. They will become clearer with practice.

Once you have visualized the person, passively experience any feelings, emotions, and memories that might come up. It is common with some people in your life to experience memories that you otherwise wouldn't typically remember. For example, I have visualized my father who passed away when I was fifteen years old. Since this happened many decades ago and he died traumatically, I repressed many memories of the times we spent together. During the visualization training I remembered moments that I had stored away in my subconscious.

For people who are currently in your life, you may have certain questions that you want answers to. At this stage we can promote alterations in our perceptions of these significant people. At deep levels of this training I have found the experience to be similar to the experience of dreams that feel completely real while experiencing them. Many people engaged in this training are surprised at the number of revelations that come to the surface. These revelations help us to deal with unresolved issues in our relationships with those we choose to visualize, or on the flip side, help us to strengthen our bond with those we love.

+ Choose specific people to visualize in your session; write down their names beforehand if you wish.
+ Perform a good standard AT session, but don't cancel at the end.
+ Now concentrate on the middle of your forehead for a few moments, then gently move your eyes inward, then upward toward your third eye.
+ Maintain your passive AT state for twenty to thirty minutes and begin to visualize the first person.
+ Visualize a few more persons on your list, canceling as described in training #12 between each person and at the end of your session.

Training #14
Visualization of Abstract Concepts

Visualization of an abstract concept seems like a rather novel idea. How can we visualize a concept? Well, it is possible—it's all about internalizing the specific concept we want to visualize. Sometimes the concepts can come to mind as words do on a printed page. Other times they come as more of an acoustic experience. They can also come as a bodily experience. The most important feature of this is not so much how you get there but what it is you are thinking about. Abstract concepts such as freedom, justice, or happiness have to do mostly with the bigger life situations we find ourselves in. How do you feel about those situations of life? How about peace, love, anger, or prejudice?

All of us have our own unique life story and situations that affect us the most. Ask yourself about the above life situations and how they pertain to you. What other life situations affect you? In this visualization you bring to light the feeling of the word(s) that describes the abstract situation (in whatever way is most effective for you). Then you simply "sit back" and passively watch what happens. You may get in touch with certain feelings, sometimes very deeply, or you may start to visualize scenes, static pictures, images, or symbols. Whatever crosses your mind's eye, simply let it in and accept whatever form in which the concept manifests. Allow yourself the freedom to explore this manifestation however and wherever it takes you. If for whatever reason you feel you have gone too far, cancel immediately. During the course of this book you will find many trainings that may bolster your feelings and attitudes toward these abstract concepts in a positive direction.

+ Choose specific concepts to visualize in your session; write them down if you wish.
+ Perform a good standard AT session, but don't cancel at the end.
+ Now concentrate on the middle of your forehead for a few moments, then gently move your eyes inward, then upward toward your third eye.
+ Maintain your passive AT state for twenty to thirty minutes and begin to visualize your first concept. Visualize others one at a time and passively watch where each one takes you.
+ Cancel as described in training #12 between each concept and at the end of your session.

Training #15
Self-Participation and Selected States of Feeling

This training involves selected states of feeling where we passively participate in our visualization. Wolfgang Luthe explains: "During this phase of meditative training, the trainee gradually learns to experience a psychophysiological state which is in correspondence with his meditative intention. During prolonged training periods (thirty to sixty minutes), passive concentration should focus on a specific state of overall feeling, for example, the feeling one experiences while looking over the wide and open ocean."[2]

In this training we inject ourselves into the visualization-meditation process based on real-life situations. As Luthe states, this relates to an "overall feeling" that we may experience when we call to mind a landscape or other scene that has a view. Oftentimes this can be a wide-open ocean vista as Luthe suggests, or such scenes as the view from a mountaintop, a sunrise, flying through the clouds, or seeing Earth from the vantage of the moon. It is also common to revisit a place like a house where you once lived, a cemetery, a schoolyard, or a place in nature that you hold dear.

Frequently the view unfolds in one of two ways. The first way is that you see the scene as an observer, looking at it through your own eyes. And you then feel the scene and experience the emotions it stimulates as if you were actually there. The second way is that you visualize yourself from the outside, seeing yourself acting in the scene as if you were watching a movie or looking at a picture or photograph. In both cases you will probably notice that the moving visualization you have acquired is more easily maintained than a static image. These "filmstrips" are extremely helpful in gaining insights (both pleasing and unpleasant) and can be used in resolving many situations of a psychological and physiological nature, invoking a desire for healing. Because self-generated healing toward optimum health is the goal of this book, this training is very useful toward that goal.

✦ Perform a good standard AT session, but don't cancel at the end.

✦ Now concentrate on the middle of your forehead for a few moments, then gently move your eyes inward, then upward toward your third eye.

✦ Maintain your passive AT state for twenty to thirty minutes, and then begin to visualize your scene (from either perspective mentioned above) and connect with the feelings this invokes.

✦ Visualize each scene one at a time and passively watch where each one takes you.

✦ Cancel as described in training #12 between each scene and at the end of your session.

Training #16
Using Self-Directed Questions

The final training in this chapter allows you to gain more information about yourself. This is done by asking yourself questions in a deep state of AT and then passively watching what happens. Begin by thinking of circumstances in your life you have questions about. It's important to do this before you begin this session because it is usually more difficult to come up with appropriate questions when you are already deep in an AT frame of mind (although it is possible for questions to come to you spontaneously during your AT session, and sometimes this is a good thing). So my suggestion is to be prepared, and if spontaneous questions arise during the session, then definitely pursue them.

Sometimes answers to a question come during the session, but certainly not always; regardless, you have planted the seed of your question in a deep AT state, so you will definitely come up with an answer eventually. On many occasions answers come later in the day, or the next day, or even in dreams at night.

I'm not going to suggest questions to use here in this exercise because these will be completely individual and should spring from your own personal needs or problems.

+ Choose specific self-directed questions to frame during the session, and write them down if you wish.

+ Perform a good standard AT session, but don't cancel at the end.

+ Now concentrate on the middle of your forehead for a few moments, then gently move your eyes inward, then upward toward your third eye.

+ Maintain your passive AT state for twenty to thirty minutes, and then begin to ask your first question.

+ Frame your questions one at a time and passively watch where they take you.

+ Cancel as described in training #12 between each question and at the end of your session.

I like to use this technique when I get writer's block. I'll formulate a specific question related to the book I'm writing, then I'll do an AT session (sometimes along with the scent of an essential oil—scent trainings are included in chapter 12), ask my question, and see what manifests in terms of an answer.

9

APPLYING AUTOGENIC
TRAINING TO MEDITATION
AND TO THE
SUBTLE-ENERGY CENTERS

Accounts and records of the phenomenological practices of meditation date back to well over two thousand years ago. Today we have a plethora of scientific studies regarding the psychophysiological benefits of meditation. From studying Indian yogis, Zen monks, and more recently, modern meditators in Western countries, it is quite clear that our neurophysiological processes can be altered through meditative techniques. Some of these changes include slowing of heart rate and breathing, decrease in oxygen consumption, lowering and stabilizing blood pressure, and decreased skin conductivity. EEG testing, which measures and records electric currents in the brain, shows increased alpha brain waves during deep meditation. During a deep alpha state we are completely relaxed; this is not the same as sleep, which occurs with theta brain waves. When practiced properly, you don't get drowsy during meditation; on the contrary, just like with AT, you remain fully alert and awake.

It is important to note that meditation practices, similar to AT, have many health benefits in the realm of psychosomatic medicine and autonomic functioning. Both AT and meditation induce deep relaxation, in some cases even deeper than that achieved in sleep. These deep forms of relaxation are basically the opposite of the neurophysiological patterns of stress we are bombarded with during our waking hours and even at times when sleeping, during periods of weird or bad dreams. When practiced correctly, the positive effects of AT and meditation carry through into our daily lives. Studies have shown a drop in the frequency of headaches, colds, and insomnia. Meditation practice can help people make positive dietary changes, eliminating junk foods and processed foods and increasing fresh foods. Diligent meditation practice has also been found to influence lifestyle changes, including reduced use of nicotine, alcohol, caffeine, and drugs, whether prescription or recreational.

From my own work with clients it is clear that meditation is most effective for people who have a positive attitude toward the practice—a fact supported by scientific research. There are some people who have a negative predisposition toward meditation and see it as a sort of mystical escapism. Unless they are convinced otherwise they will most likely not be successful with meditative techniques. Those of us with a positive predisposition toward meditation will be much more likely to take the time to practice diligently and add in the philosophical components, thereby experiencing the cumulative benefits.

As you will see as we progress through this chapter, we will be using our experience thus far with AT in combination with meditation. This is a powerful and remarkable combination of psychophysiological techniques: the standard AT formulas, visualization (advanced AT) formulas, and meditation. In addition, the meditative component will be added to AT in a novel way—by accessing the ethereal body and the chakras, which I refer to as *energetic tunnels* (more on this later in this chapter).

It is important to note that just because someone can meditate effectively doesn't make him a better person. With the rise in popularity of meditation and a host of other personal-growth modalities, I have seen over the last two decades a sort of "superiority complex" arise among certain people, including meditators. It has become very popular now to participate in human-potential groups and movements, personal-growth seminars, quasireligious mind-control modalities, and ersatz Native American ceremonies led by non–Native Americans.

There are plenty of people paying big money to follow self-styled gurus. An experience with this type of thing that had personal significance happened while I was living in the amazing red rocks of Sedona, Arizona (often referred to as the New Age capital of the world). Just a few miles away from my house there was (and still is) a picturesque retreat center called Angel Valley. In October 2009, self-help guru James Arthur Ray rented the center for his "Spiritual Warrior" retreat, which lasted several days and cost participants over $9,000. Ray is a middle-age Caucasian man who uses many Native American ceremonies. During the course of this retreat he had people fast while on a thirty-six-hour vision quest in the Arizona desert in which participants said he "played God."[1] Then on day five he crammed more than sixty people into a sweat lodge measuring just 415 square feet and covered with plastic. Authentic Native American sweat lodges restrict the number of people to however many can sit against the outside wall of the lodge. In my experience this is usually between ten and twenty people depending on the size of the lodge. Native Americans also never use plastic to cover a sweat lodge—it's just not safe, as the melting plastic is highly toxic and holds too much heat in without letting air circulate. James Ray's lodge heated up to the point where people started vomiting and passing out. Witnesses say Ray shouted at them to "push through it."[2] In the end, three people died and eighteen were hospitalized after suffering burns, dehydration, breathing problems, kidney failure, or elevated body temperature. Afterward, one participant reported that when the EMTs arrived Ray didn't even help: "He didn't do anything, he didn't participate in helping. He did nothing. He just stood there."[3]

Ray didn't stick around; he immediately went on to lead two more scheduled retreats in Los Angeles and San Diego. He was finally arrested in February 2010, found guilty on three counts of federal negligent homicide, and sentenced to two years in prison. After this tragedy, our small community in Sedona was devastated. Sedona is surrounded by Native American reservations and tribal lands where the sacred sweat lodge is practiced. Many of my Yavapai, Hualapai, and Havasupai friends and mentors were both sad and outraged, but they also took time to educate people about the sweat lodge and the proper way to conduct a lodge ceremony.

I bring up this example because it shows the blind faith some people can have when dealing with subjects of personal growth, spirituality, and religion. We often also put blind faith in our medical practitioners. In the case of the followers of self-appointed gurus, of which there are hundreds like James Ray, and followers of many of the human-potential movements and groups, we can clearly see a complex where belonging to the guru or the group becomes even more important than the benefits of the teachings.

In this portion of the training we are addressing techniques of meditation. Meditation and working with the ethereal or subtle body is a central part of more than a few major religions, including Hindu tantra, Buddhist tantra, Bon, Qigong, and Hesychasm, to name a few. But in this case we are not attaching any religious or spiritual context to our work. We are involved here in *self-generated* training—no gurus, priests, masters, or whatever. In a nutshell, all of our AT and PM trainings and techniques are highly individual personal practices. You alone are responsible for your own practice. There is no place in this kind of practice for a superiority complex.

THE SUBTLE BODY AND ENERGY TUNNELS

The subtle body is also known as "the most sacred body," "the true and genuine body," "the diamond body," "the light body," "the rainbow body," "the body of bliss," and "the immortal body" in various schools of Eastern thought and mysticism. It can be described as an energy matrix that, yes, actually exists even though we normally can't see it, much like radio waves, which we can't measure or see, or the waves that connect our cell phones and computers. We know those forms of energy exist because we can feel the results of working with them, and in the case of radios, cell phones, and computers, we certainly know we can use them. Some masters of Buddhism, Taoism, Sufism, and Hermeticism, to name a few, as well as some psychic-aura readers, claim to be able to actually see the subtle-energy body; they say that it is located between a quarter of an inch to two inches out from our physical body and is attached to the physical body at seven main chakras or *energy tunnels* (my term).* Most us have to make do with experiencing the subtle-energy body and the energy tunnels by intentionally working with them.

Before we move on to the trainings, I'd like to introduce some scientific proof for the subtle-energy or etheric body and the energy tunnels for the skeptics among us. Let's begin with researcher and medical doctor Richard Gerber. In his classic book on the subject *Vibrational Energy,* Dr. Gerber states:

> There is considerable evidence to suggest that there exists a holographic energy template associated with the physical body. This etheric (subtle) body is a body which looks quite similar to the physical body over which it is superimposed. Within the energetic map is carried information which guides the cellular growth of the physical structure of the body. It carries special information on how the developing fetus is to unfold in utero, and also structural data for growth and repair of the adult organism should damage or disease occur. This energetic structure works in concert with the cellular genetic mechanisms that molecular biology has elabo-

---

*Chakra is from the Sanskrit word for "wheel" or "turning." Many people use this term, but I prefer *energy tunnel* because it describes this form of subtle energy perfectly and because I don't speak Sanskrit. And so in this book I use that term.

rated upon over the last several decades of medical research. The physical body is so energetically connected and dependent upon the etheric body for cellular guidance that the physical body cannot exist without the etheric body. If the etheric field becomes distorted, physical disease follows. Many illnesses begin first in the etheric body and then are later manifested in the physical body as organ pathology.[4]

Hiroshi Motoyama, a Japanese parapsychologist, scientist, spiritual instructor, and author, has presented his experimental findings on the presence of the chakra system in human beings. Dr. Motoyama created a special lead-lined recording booth electrically shielded from outside electromagnetic disturbance. A movable copper electrode was positioned opposite the various chakras of the people being tested, many of whom were advanced meditators. When the electrode was placed in front of a chakra that the subject claimed to awaken or connect to, the amplitude and frequency of the electric field over the chakra was significantly greater than the energy recorded from the corresponding chakra of control subjects. In this study certain people could consciously project energy through their chakras. This phenomenon was replicated many times in Dr. Motoyama's lab over the course of a number of years of testing.[5] Dr. Motoyama's findings were duplicated by Itzhak Bentov, a researcher of physiological changes associated with meditation, using similar equipment.

In the 1970s, Valerie Hunt, a research scientist, author, lecturer, and professor emeritus of physiological science at UCLA best known for her pioneering research in the field of bioenergy, conducted research on the energetic and therapeutic effects of the physical manipulative technique known as Rolfing. But what she found instead had more to do with the chakra system. Using EMG electrodes (usually used to measure the electrical potential of muscles), she studied bioelectrical energy variations in areas of the skin corresponding to the positions of the chakras. What she found were regular, high-frequency, sinusoidal electrical oscillations coming from these points that had never previously been recorded nor reported in the scientific literature. Dr. Hunt then had a well-known "psychic observer" of auric fields, Rosalyn Bruyere, make observations of a subject's energetic field while the chakras were being electronically monitored. During her observations, Bruyere was not given feedback as to the activities of the EMG electrodes attached to the chakra points. Unexpectedly, Dr. Hunt found that Bruyere's auric observations, which related to color changes in the subject's energetic field, correlated *exactly* with the EMG electrode recordings. Dr. Hunt discovered that each color of the aura was associated with a different wave pattern recorded at the chakra points of her subjects. The wave patterns were then named after the auric colors they were found to be associated with. When Bruyere described red in a subject's aura, she didn't know it but the EMG displayed and recorded the wave pattern associated with red. This was also proven with other colors.[6]

What Are Energy Tunnels?

The seven main energy tunnels, also referred to as *energy vortices, power centers,* and the more common term, *chakras,* are energy centers that connect specific points in the subtle-energy body with specific areas within the physical body. Rotating vortices of subtle-energy matter, these energy tunnels are considered focal points for the reception and transmission of energies. They also have psychological components that we will experience during these trainings. As popular author and teacher Caroline Myss (www.myss.com) famously states:

> There are seven power centers in your body, called chakras. The state of each chakra reflects the health of a particular area of your body. It also reflects your psychological, emotional and spiritual well-being. Every thought and experience you've ever had in your life gets filtered through these chakra databases. Each event is recorded into your cells. In other words, "your biography becomes your biology."

The seven main energy tunnels are located along the spinal column, from the base of the spine to the top of the head. Some systems also list numerous other smaller or minor energy centers or chakras that exist throughout the physical and subtle-energy body. For our training we are going to work only with the seven main energy tunnels, using AT, visualization, and meditation. Each energy tunnel has its own distinctive qualities and energy that correspond to specific areas of the body and functions of consciousness. Table 9.1 (page 90) provides an overview of the general characteristics of each of the seven main energy tunnels:

One way to relate to the energy tunnels is to imagine them as doors that open into separate worlds that are all connected. For example, imagine that you are standing before seven closed doors; however, instead of the doors all being on the same level they are arranged one above another, with a spiral staircase connecting the different levels. If you were to open any of the doors and enter the world within, your experiences, way of thinking, emotional state, and way of relating to others would be entirely different from what they would be were you to ascend or descend the staircase and cross the threshold of any other doorway and into another world. This is analogous to the different modes of consciousness of the seven energetic tunnels.

Notice that the colors of the energy tunnels are the exact same colors and in the same order as the colors of the rainbow, from red at the base to violet/white at the crown. Our bodies are literally walking rainbows! If you hold a crystal up to sunlight it displays beautiful vibrant rainbows that can give you an idea of what a healthy, happy human energy system looks like. Color is absorbed physiologically by the eyes, skin, and skull and energetically by our subtle body and into our energy tunnels. For these trainings we are going to use our color visualization skills in conjunction with AT and meditation to enhance our ability to enter the energy tunnels. Color is simply light of varying wavelengths; thus each color has its own particular wavelength and energy. Each tunnel color has its own feeling, traits, aspects, specific areas of the body, and functions of consciousness.

TABLE 9.1. GENERAL CHARACTERISTICS OF THE ENERGY TUNNELS

Energy Tunnel	Center of	Location	Color	Element	Gland(s)	Sense
1. Base	survival	base of spine	red	earth	adrenals	smell
2. Sacral	emotions	pelvis	orange	water	reproductive	taste
3. Solar Plexus	power	solar plexus	yellow	fire	pancreas	sight
4. Heart	connection	center of chest	green	air	thymus	touch
5. Throat	communication	throat	sky blue	sound	thyroid	hearing
6. Brow	intuition	behind forehead	indigo blue	light	pituitary	intuition
7. Crown	enlightenment	top of head	violet or white	thought	pineal	n/a

Making Your Own Color Fields

To begin, we will work with meditation on a specific color. To do this properly I'm going to share with you a little secret that will take a bit of time and effort but is well worth it. When I first began working with colors I took a color-therapy course, which was very enlightening. However, even though the information was good I was disappointed because I never really got into the colors and feelings/meanings. I thought maybe it was just me or that I was doing it wrong. The instructor had us using colored sheets of paper to focus on, and she also had objects of the colors of the rainbow such as statuettes (mostly animals), small pieces of colored fabric, and colored pencils. She gave us sheets of colored paper to take home with us to practice.

During the next few days I practiced meditating on the colored sheets of paper, but I still wasn't getting it until I finally realized one important thing: my mind was not focusing solely on the color because of all the other things I could see around the edges of the paper with my peripheral vision. As an avid outdoorsman, rock climber, and when younger an experienced hunter, my mind over many decades has been trained to see and hear everything that's going on around me (which sometimes other people find a bit annoying). The next day I went to a store that sold fabric and purchased a large piece of red cloth. I held it up in front me, close to my face, so that almost all of my peripheral vision was blocked, and *voila!* All I could see was red. Later that day I tried the meditation using my big piece of red cloth; I finally found the secret that I'm about to share with you here.

Now for those of you who don't know this—and I certainly didn't— fabric is typically sold by the yard. While a yard of fabric is always 36" long, the fabric on a bolt (the way it comes rolled up to the store) can vary anywhere from 32" to 60" in width on average. Therefore, a measured yard of fabric is not a 36" square (unless you purchase a yard of 36"-width fabric, which is an uncommon width). I have found that the most common widths are 45" and 60" inches. So if you purchase a yard, it will most likely measure either 45" or 60" in width. A single yard of solid cloth should be plenty unless you are a very tall person. My ideal size is approximately 33" by 41", which easily fits into one typical yard of fabric. When I buy a yard of fabric that is 45" wide I either ask to have it cut to the size I want where I bought it or cut it myself at home. The length is not as important as the width. You can easily hold a piece of fabric that is a little too wide, but it's more comfortable to just cut it to your proper size. To determine your size, follow these simple instructions:

How to Make Your Own Color Field

+ Get a tape measure.
+ Pull the tape out in front of you at eye level, three or four inches from the tip of your nose.
+ Extend the tape out with your arms while looking straight ahead. Continue extending the tape out until you can barely see your hands with your peripheral vision while keeping the tape at eye level.
+ Note on the tape how many inches you have extended it. That will be the proper width for your cloth.
+ Now measure from about four inches above your head down to a couple of inches below your belt line or belly button.
+ If your dimensions are smaller than a typical yard of fabric either 46" or 60" wide, just purchase one yard and cut it to your dimensions. An alternate way is to purchase a yard first and measure yourself with the actual fabric in the way just described, and then cut it.

I have found solid colors of fabric to be fairly inexpensive, usually between $5 and $10 a yard. It's not necessary to buy all seven colors at once. I like to try a yard of a specific fabric first to see if I like it. The main thing is to buy a piece that is more opaque than see-through and try it out before you buy more colors. The first color we will be working with is red, so purchase that piece first. As you will see, during this training we will be holding the colored fabric in front of our eyes for short periods of time. For people uncomfortable with this or for those who just want to try something different than meditating with colored fabric, here is another option:

There are a few companies (easy to find online or order through an office-supply store if they don't carry them) that make cardboard trifold presentation board. You can buy one for less than $10. They also make them in foam, which is a little more rigid, for a few dollars more. The usual size is 48" wide by 36" high, which is ideal for most people sitting on the floor for these exercises. Basically, it's just a piece of cardboard 48" wide, with a fold 12" in from either side, and a height of 36", so that when folded together it becomes 24" wide by 36" high. What you do with this in our color work is stand it up with the 12" "wings" only partially folded in, at a 45-degree angle or so. You sit right in front of the 24" main section to do your meditating. The side wings prevent your peripheral vision from distracting you, and you don't have to hold a cloth up, as in the first option. You will still need to purchase colored cloth and drape it over the board because the trifold display boards only come in a few colors. For work with special-needs clients I have purchased the brand Spotlight in black for $5. There are other companies, such as Pacon, that make the trifold board as well.

Although I prefer fabric, another economical alternative is colored poster board or colored construction paper. Packs of colored poster board usually don't have all the colors, but you could use the ones they have and substitute colored paper for the others. The typical size is 22" by 28", and they usually come twenty-five sheets to a package for around $20. However, you can buy a 200-sheet pack of 9" by 12" construction paper specifically with the seven colors of the rainbow for around $5. In either case take your measurements as described above, and then simply tape the pieces of paper together with some shipping tape to the proper size.

In the following exercises I will describe using a cloth, but if you use a trifold presentation board that you sit in front of and that wraps around your field of vision, you won't have to hold a cloth up for fifteen minutes, which is a whole lot easier on the arms.

Training #17
First Tunnel—Red

Associated organs/body parts: kidneys and bladder, the vertebral column, hips, legs

Associated gland: adrenal glands

Associated problems: constipation, diarrhea, piles, colitis,
Crohn's disease, cold fingers and toes, frequency of urination,
hypertension (high blood pressure), kidney stones, impotence,
hip problems, problems of the legs and feet

Personality traits: courage, confidence, humanism, strength of
will, spontaneity, honesty, extroversion

Positive aspects of red: security, courage, strength of will, pioneering spirit

Negative aspects of red: insecurity, self-pitying, aggression, fear

The color red governs the first energy tunnel situated at the base of the
spine. This is a powerful energy storage area that when released by life-
or-death situations or certain meditations and body manipulations rises
up the spine, activating all the other energy tunnels before rushing out
the top of the head. In some traditions such as the Hindu, this energy
release, called a *kundalini experience* or *kundalini rising,* is much sought
after by shamans, yogis, and healers.

For us, the quality and vitality we feel while looking into this first
energy tunnel can be a strong indicator of the basic health of our entire
human organism. At a psychological level this tunnel and its red color
relate to primal self-awareness, survival, stability, and our place on the
earth. Memories stored here often include childhood traumas, physical
accidents and illnesses, and near-death experiences. On the flip side we
also carry in this tunnel our deep, primal connection to the grounded-
ness of the earth's energy. When we can connect to these energies of the
first tunnel, we tend to feel safe and secure.

+ Once you have your red meditation fabric (which I will hereafter refer to as a *drape*), board, or paper, get into a comfortable meditative AT position such as the yoga half-lotus. Simply sitting on the floor with your legs crossed is fine too; the main thing is to be in a comfortable position to view the color field in front of you.

+ Begin by closing your eyes, using the *I breathe me* formula just like all other AT sessions. After about two minutes of *I breathe me* passive breathing, open your eyes and hold your red drape in front of you, close to the tip of your nose. Spread your arms the entire width of the drape. If you measured correctly, your elbows should be extended horizontally out farther than your shoulders, so that the drape covers all or most of your peripheral vision. The portion of your arms between your elbows and shoulders should be horizontal to the floor or a tiny bit higher. The idea is to have your hands at the level of the top of your head or slightly higher and your arms comfortably extended just far enough so that all you see is red.

+ Focus on red with all of your being. Internalize it while also concentrating on the base of your spine. Breathe normally and keep developing this meditative state for at least fifteen minutes or for however much time is comfortable so that you internalize red. If your arms feel tired, close your eyes, lay the drape in your lap, keep red in your mind, and after a minute or two resume holding the drape as before.

+ Once you have fully internalized red, close your eyes and lay the drape in your lap.

+ With your eyes closed, keep the color red in your mind's eye.

+ Now place the fingers of both hands on the bone at the very base of your spine, which is at the top of your butt cheeks, and perform AT using formulas related to the first tunnel. You can use just first-tunnel formulas by silently repeating them, or mix them in with standard formulas. I prefer the latter. Examples of these formulas include:

    My base is red and warm.

    I feel my primal connection to the earth.

    The root of my being is balanced.

    My adrenaline is properly balanced and ready for action.

✦ Once you have finished with your physiological AT experience, perform psychological formulas by asking yourself simple questions related to the base tunnel. Passively wait for the answers to come. Use the above descriptions of the base tunnel and the color red to formulate your questions. Examples include:

> *What do I do to survive?* (For us modern people, a large part of this answer usually comes in a way related to how we make a living and our personal relationships.)
>
> *What are my core strengths?*
>
> *Do I feel secure in my current life?*
>
> *Do I feel powerful and assertive?* (If not, ask *How can I become more assertive?*)
>
> *What I am afraid of?*
>
> *What can I do to become more secure in my life?*
>
> *What grounds me?*

✦ These are just suggestions. As you continue practicing this training and you continue to connect deeper to your base tunnel and the color red you will naturally find that questions and answers come spontaneously.

✦ When you are ready, pick up your drape and hold it in front of you the same way as before, then open your eyes and focus on red until it is fully internalized once again. This could be almost immediately or might take a minute or two. Don't rush the process.

✦ End your session with an affirmation while staying "in the red" with eyes open. Say your affirmation to the red and your base tunnel out loud. Some examples include:

> *I have the right to be me, just as I am.*
>
> *I am connected to my body.*
>
> *I am connected to the earth.*
>
> *I am safe.*
>
> *I am centered.*
>
> *I am grounded.*
>
> *My energy resonates with balance, vitality, strength, security, trust, abundance, and prosperity.*

If you feel you have fully engaged with this red training, carry it with you and move on to the second tunnel. If you feel you need more practice, that's great too—the more you practice, the better. There is no time limit here. Enjoy, be happy, and know that by engaging in these trainings you are proactively nurturing your entire psychophysiological being toward optimum health.

Training #18

Second Tunnel—Orange

Associated organs: uterus, large intestine, prostate

Associated glands: ovaries and testes (In a fetus the testes develop in the lower abdomen, thus linking with the second energy tunnel, then descend to the scrotum at birth.)

Associated problems: premenstrual syndrome, problems with menstrual flow, uterine fibroids, ovarian cysts, irritable bowel syndrome, endometriosis, testicular disease, prostate disease

Personality traits: enthusiasm, happiness, sociability, energy, sportiness, self-assurance, constructiveness

Positive aspects of orange: sociability, creativity, joy, independence

Negative aspects of orange: withdrawal, destructiveness, despondency, overdependence

---

The second energy tunnel is an orange vortex situated in the lower abdomen and pelvic region. The basic functions of this tunnel are raw emotion, reproduction, fertility, sexual attraction, and sexual energy in general. It is also the center of creativity, from the creation of new life in the womb to the creation of characters on a page, a work of art, or an entire symphony. It is also here that information comes forward quite often about your relationship with your mother or father, your partner, or your children. Structural anomalies or energy blockages in this part of the body typically affect your attitudes toward sexuality and govern how you relate to your sexual partners. They can also block creative flow. Often, so-called writer's block can be traced to changes in flow of the second energy tunnel.

Orange is the color of success and relates to self-respect; having the ability to give ourselves the freedom to be ourselves helps us expand our interests and activities, brings joy to our work, and strengthens our appetite for life. The energy induced by the color orange is a great emotional stimulant. It connects us to our senses and helps remove inhibitions, making us independent and more social.

+ Once you have your orange-colored meditation fabric, board, or paper, get into a meditative AT position such as the yoga half-lotus. Simply sitting on the floor with your legs crossed is fine too; the main thing is to be in a comfortable position to view the color field in front of you.

+ Begin by closing your eyes, silently saying *I breathe me* as in all the other AT sessions. After about two minutes of this passive breathing, open your eyes and hold your orange drape in front of you close to the tip of your nose.

+ Focus on orange with all of your being. Internalize it while also concentrating on your lower abdomen. Breathe normally and keep developing this meditative state for at least fifteen minutes or for however much time is comfortable for you to internalize orange. If your arms feel tired, close your eyes, lay the drape in your lap, keep orange in your mind, and after a minute or two resume holding the drape.

+ Once you have fully internalized orange, close your eyes and lay the drape in your lap.

+ With your eyes closed, keep the color orange in your mind's eye.

+ Now place your hands on your lower abdomen, between your belly button and genitals, and perform AT using formulas related to the second energy tunnel. You can use second-tunnel formulas alone, silently repeating them, or mix them in with standard formulas. I prefer the latter. Some examples:

> *My lower abdomen is warm.*
> *My ovaries (or testes) are mystical manifestations of creation.*
> *My bowels are calm and regular.*
> *My gut feels healthy and strong.*

+ Once you have finished with your physiological AT experience, perform psychological formulas by silently asking yourself simple questions related to the second energy tunnel, passively waiting for the answers. Use the above descriptions of the second energy tunnel and the color orange to formulate your questions. Examples include:

> *How do I deal with my raw emotions?*
>
> *What kind of person am I sexually attracted to?*
>
> *What have I created lately?*
>
> *What do I want to create?*
>
> *Do I give myself enough freedom to do what I want to do?*
>
> *What new interests or activities do I want to pursue?*
>
> *How can I make my work more enjoyable?*
>
> *What is my relationship with . . .* (mother, father, siblings, et al.)*?*

✦ When you feel finished with your questions/answers, pick up your drape and hold it in front of you the same way as before, then open your eyes and focus on orange until it is fully internalized once again. This could be almost immediately or might take a minute or two. Don't rush the process.

✦ End your session with an affirmation while staying "in the orange" with eyes open. Say it out loud to the orange and to your second tunnel. Some sample affirmations:

> *I have the right to feel my own feelings.*
>
> *I am enough.*
>
> *I have enough.*
>
> *I am passionate.*
>
> *I am adaptable.*
>
> *I enjoy, value, and respect my body.*
>
> *I am creative.*
>
> *My energy resonates with enthusiasm, harmony, nurturance, and pleasure.*

Training #19
Third Tunnel—Yellow

Associated organs: liver, spleen, stomach, and small intestine
Associated gland: pancreas

Associated problems: diabetes, pancreatitis, liver disease, peptic ulcer, celiac disease, gallstones

Personality traits: good humor, optimism, confidence, practicality, intellectualness

Positive aspects of yellow: confidence, alertness, optimism, good humor

Negative aspects of yellow: feelings of inferiority, overanalysis, sarcasm, pessimism

---

The third energy tunnel relates to the solar plexus, and its color is yellow. It is located between the bottom of the sternum and the belly button. This tunnel generates action, assertion, and power and often reveals to us personal patterns related to our power and our misconceptions and obstacles in using our power. The power associated with the third energy tunnel provides us with leadership skills; we can command audiences, and we are generally noticeable by others. Entertainers, community leaders, teachers, and other high-profile people usually have very strong yellow tunnel energy. The yellow tunnel also relates to self-worth—how we feel about ourselves and how we feel others perceive us. This is the area of the personality, the ego, and the intellect, and it is associated with self-confidence.

At the physiological level the third tunnel relates to the complex functioning of the pancreas. The pancreas makes pancreatic juices and hormones, including insulin and secretin. Pancreatic juices contain enzymes that help digest food in the small intestine. Both pancreatic enzymes and hormones are needed to keep the body functioning correctly. The third energy tunnel acts as a sort of generator and monitors energy distribution throughout the entire body. When this tunnel is not functioning optimally we tend to feel tired, listless, and withdrawn. Self-monitoring the third tunnel is especially important during and after times when we are especially assertive, when we exert high volumes of physical energy, or when we are feeling powerless or inhibited.

✦ Once you have your yellow-colored meditation fabric, board, or paper, get into a comfortable meditative AT position such as the yoga half-lotus. Simply sitting on the floor with your legs crossed is fine too; the main thing is to be in a comfortable position to view the color field in front of you.

✦ Begin by closing your eyes and silently saying *I breathe me* as in all the other AT sessions. After about two minutes of this passive breathing, open your eyes and hold your yellow drape in front of you close to the tip of your nose.

✦ Focus on yellow with all your being. Internalize it while also concentrating on the area of your solar plexus. Breathe normally, and keep developing this meditative state for at least fifteen minutes or for however much time is comfortable in order to internalize yellow. If your arms feel tired, close your eyes, lay the drape in your lap, keep yellow in your mind, and after a minute or two, resume holding the drape.

✦ Once you have fully internalized yellow, close your eyes and lay the drape in your lap.

✦ With your eyes closed, keep the color yellow in your mind's eye.

✦ Now place your hands on your solar plexus and perform AT using formulas related to the third energy tunnel. You can use just use third-tunnel formulas by silently repeating them, or mix them in with standard formulas. I prefer the latter. Some examples:

> *My solar plexus is warm.*
> *My digestion is calm and healthy.*
> *My energy distribution is even and vigorous.*
> *My energetic body feels strong and positive.*

✦ Once you have finished with your physiological AT experience, perform psychological formulas by silently asking yourself simple questions related to the third energy tunnel, passively waiting for the answers. Use the above descriptions of the third tunnel and the color yellow to formulate your questions. Some examples:

> *How do I assert myself physically?*
> *How do I assert myself mentally?*
> *Am I optimistic of the future?*
> *Do I feel confident?*

How do I feel speaking in front of people?

Do I have any personal patterns I want or need to change?

✦ When you feel finished with your questions/answers, pick up your drape and hold it in front of you the same way as before, then open your eyes and focus on yellow until it is fully internalized once again. This could be almost immediately or might take a minute or two. Don't rush the process.

✦ End your session with an affirmation while staying "in the yellow" with eyes open. Say the affirmation out loud to the yellow and to your solar plexus tunnel. Some examples:

I am courageous.

I can meet any challenge.

I am free to act, choose, grow, and heal.

I am capable.

I stand up for myself and what I believe in.

My energy resonates with confidence, purpose, warmth, and joy.

Training #20
Fourth Tunnel—Green

Associated organs: heart and breasts

Associated gland: thymus gland

Associated problems: heart diseases, high blood pressure, allergies, breast cancer, diseases and problems of the immune system

Personality traits: understanding, self-control, adaptability, sympathy, compassion, generosity, humility, love of nature, romance

Positive aspects of green: compassion, generosity, harmony/balance, love

Negative aspects of green: indifference, jealousy, miserliness, bitterness

The fourth energy tunnel is a green vortex located in the area of the heart. For most people of our culture this tunnel is probably the most noticed and worked on simply because it is the seat of love in all its variations: self-love, love of others, acceptance, emotion, intimacy. It also concerns all those situations that go along with love when it goes haywire. The heart tunnel is like the brain of our emotional self. "Thinking with our heart" instead of "thinking with our head" is something we have all probably experienced more than once.

In terms of the energy tunnels, the heart tunnel is a transmitting station between the lower energy tunnels (red, orange, and yellow) and the upper tunnels (blue, indigo, and violet). It's important to realize that *lower* and *upper,* in this context, are simply descriptive words and have no bearing on importance of functioning. Some people mistakenly believe that the upper energy tunnels are somehow superior to the lower ones, and that the goal of personal growth via our energy tunnels is to process through the lower ones in order to focus and remain in the upper tunnels. Nothing could be further from the truth. Each energy center serves a vitally important function within the whole system, and growth is facilitated through each tunnel. If you attempt to live only through the upper chakras you create an imbalance that can impede growth and health. Plus, the fact is that we wouldn't be alive if it weren't for our first-tunnel adrenals, our second-tunnel reproductive organs, and our third-tunnel pancreas.

Physiologically, we all know that the heart pumps blood, and that a healthy heart is vitally important. The inner workings of the heart are complex, and there's no point on elaborating them here. However, in my personal research of how the heart functions I discovered many amazing things, and I recommend that everyone learn more about this remarkable organ and what it does for us at a deeper level. One fairly simple fact about the heart that I previously was unaware of—which relates to this training—is that the heart actually has two separate but connected circulatory systems. *Pulmonary circulation* refers to the portion of the cardiovascular system that carries deoxygenated blood away from the heart to the lungs and returns oxygenated (oxygen-rich) blood back to the heart. *Systemic circulation* refers to that part of the cardiovascular system that carries oxygenated blood away from the heart to the body and returns deoxygenated blood back to the heart. We can easily correlate these two actions to receiving emotions as a result of certain situations, and then releasing emotions, as in crying, laughing, hugging, and screaming and yelling.

✦ Once you have your green-colored meditation fabric, board, or paper, get into a comfortable meditative AT position such as the yoga half-lotus. Simply sitting on the floor with your legs crossed is fine too; the main thing is to be in a comfortable position to view the color field in front of you.

✦ Begin by closing your eyes, silently saying *I breathe me* as in all the other AT sessions. After about two minutes of this passive breathing, open your eyes and hold your green drape in front of you close to the tip of your nose.

✦ Focus on green with all your being. Internalize it while also concentrating on the area of your heart, just behind and slightly left of the breastbone. Breathe normally and keep developing this meditative state for at least fifteen minutes or for however much time is comfortable in order for you to internalize green. If your arms feel tired, close your eyes, lay the drape in your lap, keep green in your mind, and after a minute or two, resume.

✦ Once you have fully internalized green, close your eyes and lay the drape in your lap.

✦ With your eyes closed, keep the color green in your mind's eye.

✦ Now place your hands on your heart and perform AT using formulas related to the fourth energy tunnel. You can just use fourth-tunnel formulas by silently repeating them, or mix them in with standard formulas. I prefer the latter. Some examples:

> *My heartbeat is calm and strong.* (Just for this formula place your index and middle finger on the jugular vein on one side of your neck and find your pulse.)
>
> *My heart is pumping nutrients throughout my body.*
>
> *My heart is pumping nasty waste to be released.*
>
> *My heart together with my lungs connects me to the green world with oxygen and CO_2.*
>
> *My heart keeps my temperature even and comfortable.*
>
> *My flowing blood is filled with disease fighters to keep away foreign invaders.*
>
> *My blood is flowing through my brain, granting the miracle of consciousness.*

✦ Once you have finished with your physiological AT experience, perform psychological formulas by silently asking yourself simple questions related to the fourth energy tunnel, passively waiting for answers. Use the above descriptions of the fourth tunnel and the color green to formulate your questions. Some examples:

> *Whom do I love?*
>
> *How do I express love to others?*
>
> *How do I express love of myself?*
>
> *What emotions do I experience the most?*
>
> *How do I express intimacy with . . . (name of significant other if you have one, or the names of your children)?*
>
> *When do I think with my heart and not my head?*

✦ When you feel finished with your questions/answers, pick up your drape and hold it in front of you the same way as before, then open your eyes and focus on green until it is fully internalized once again. This could be almost immediately or might take a minute or two. Don't rush the process.

✦ End your session with an affirmation while staying "in the green" with eyes open. Say it out loud to the green of your heart tunnel. Some examples:

> *I am a channel for divine love.*
>
> *I accept and love myself.*
>
> *I am filled with gratitude.*
>
> *I am forgiving of myself and others.*
>
> *My energy resonates with compassion, love, acceptance, and kindness.*

Training #21
Fifth Tunnel—Blue

Associated organs/body parts: throat, lungs

Associated gland: thyroid gland, upper digestive tract

Associated problems: thyroid problems (such as those listed above), anorexia nervosa (this is a multitunnel problem but has a strong connection to the throat tunnel), asthma, bronchitis, hearing problems, tinnitus; may also be connected to problems with the brow chakra, problems of the upper digestive tract, mouth ulcers, sore throat, tonsillitis

Personality traits: loyalty, tact, affection, inspiration, inventiveness, care, caution

Positive aspects of blue: loyalty, trustworthiness, tactfulness, calm

Negative aspects of blue: fickleness, unreliability, self-righteousness, coldness

---

Located in the area around the Adam's apple is the fifth energetic tunnel of sky blue. It is the tunnel of self-expression, speech, communication, and the ability to communicate our needs and requirements. Nonstop talkers and those who carry on incessantly about things that irritate them or those who just tend to dominate any setting they occupy have excess energy flowing through this tunnel. On the other hand, people who are overly shy, who don't stick up for themselves, or who can't express what they want or need have a tunnel blockage here and are deficient in this blue energy.

At the physiological level the blue tunnel is the home of the thyroid, a butterfly-shaped gland that sits low on the front of the neck, below your Adam's apple, along the front of the windpipe. The thyroid has two side lobes connected by a bridge (isthmus) in the middle. When the thyroid is normal size you can't feel it. The thyroid produces thyroid hormone (TH), which regulates, among other things, the body's temperature, metabolism, and heartbeat. Things can start to go wrong when your thyroid is under- or overactive. If it's sluggish, it produces too little TH and you're tired; amped-up and it produces too much and you're wired. What causes your thyroid to go out of balance? It could be genetics, an autoimmune attack, pregnancy, stress, nutritional deficiencies, or toxins in the environment. Because thyroid hormones roam throughout the body, from the brain to the bowels, diagnosing a thyroid disorder can be challenging. Women are as much as ten times more likely than men to have a thyroid problem, and if you're a woman over thirty-five, your odds of having a thyroid disorder are 30 percent or higher by some estimates. Most experts estimate that at least thirty million Americans have a thyroid disorder and half of them are silent sufferers who are undiagnosed.

I know of people who have been diagnosed with thyroid problems who have been greatly helped by these trainings simply because many of the situations that trigger ill health are psychosomatic, which means they involve both the mind (*psyche*) and the body (*soma*). It's a physical illness or problem caused or aggravated by a mental factor such as internal conflict or stress. Our AT, visualization, meditation, and practices of renewal of primal mind are perfect for helping to resolve internal conflict, reducing stress, and preventing illness.

Some of the symptoms associated with the thyroid, the blue energy tunnel, include exhaustion, constipation, diarrhea, depression, irregular menses, nervousness, anxiety, painful extremities and muscles, changes in appetite, high blood pressure, heart palpitations, brain fog, chills or hot flashes, diminished sex drive, changes in appetite, hoarseness, pain in neck, difficulty sleeping, dry skin, slow metabolism, weight gain.

Granted, any one of these problems could also be due to some other condition; however, these problems have been documented as being connected with either hypothyroidism (too little thyroid hormone) or hyperthyroidism (too much thyroid hormone). My point is, imbalanced thyroid conditions are extremely common in our society. If this sounds like you, do these trainings *and* go get your thyroid tested. Remember, it's always best to work with medical professionals who are concerned with your whole body, not just the current symptoms you may be experiencing and isolated body parts.

+ Once you have your blue-colored meditation fabric, board, or paper, get into a comfortable meditative AT position such as the yoga half-lotus. Simply sitting on the floor with your legs crossed is fine too; the main thing is to be in a comfortable position to view the color field in front of you.

+ Begin by closing your eyes, silently saying *I breathe me* just as in all the other AT sessions. After about two minutes of this passive breathing, open your eyes and hold your blue drape in front of you close to the tip of your nose.

+ Focus on blue with all of your being. Internalize it while also concentrating on the area of your thyroid, around your Adam's apple. Breathe normally and keep developing this meditative state for at least fifteen minutes or for however much time is comfortable in order for you to internalize blue. If your arms feel tired, close your eyes, lay the drape in your lap, keep blue in your mind, and after a minute or two resume holding the drape.

+ Once you have fully internalized blue, close your eyes and lay the drape in your lap.

+ With your eyes closed, keep the color blue in your mind's eye.

+ Now place your hands on your throat and perform AT using formulas related to the fifth energy tunnel. You can just use fifth-tunnel formulas by silently repeating them, or mix them in with standard formulas. I prefer the latter. Some examples:

> *My thyroid is regulating my body perfectly.*
> *My body temperature is comfortable and stable.*
> *My metabolic rate is healthy for my body.*
> *My heartbeat is calm and strong.*
> *My throat is clear and warm.*

+ Once you have finished with your physiological AT experience, perform psychological formulas by silently asking yourself simple questions related to the fifth energy tunnel, passively waiting for the answers. Use the above descriptions of the fifth tunnel and the color blue to formulate your questions. Some examples:

> *Am I comfortable with the way I express myself verbally?*
> *Am I effective at communicating with . . .* (names of family, friends, coworkers)?
> *Do I communicate effectively when I require or want something?*
> *What do I do when people don't give me what I deserve?*
> *What is my least effective venue for communication?*
> *How often do I not tell the truth?*
> *What can I do to express myself more effectively?*

+ When you feel finished with your questions/answers, pick up your drape and hold it in front of you the same way as before, then open your eyes and focus on blue until it is fully internalized once again. This could be almost immediately or might take a minute or two. Don't rush the process.

✦ End your session with an affirmation while staying "in the blue" with eyes open. Say it out loud to the blue and to your throat tunnel. Some examples:

I speak the truth.

I am a good listener.

I express myself with integrity.

I nourish my soul with creative expression.

I am honest.

I live an authentic life.

My communication with the world resonates with truth, honesty, and creativity.

Training #22
Sixth Tunnel—Indigo

Associated organs/body parts: eyes, lower head, sinuses

Associated gland: pituitary

Associated problems: tension headaches, migraines, sinus problems, pituitary gland tumor (These tumors are fairly common in adults. They are not brain tumors and are almost always benign—cancerous tumors of this sort are extremely rare.)

Personality traits: keen intellect, strong intuitive ability, good imagination, ability to grasp the big picture

Positive aspects of indigo: highly intuitive, faithful, sense of unity, fearlessness, devotion to duty, articulate, practical idealism

Negative aspects of indigo: isolation, fear, intolerance, impracticality, tendency to judge, inconsideration, depression

The sixth energy tunnel is located in the forehead, between and slightly above the eyebrows. It is indigo in color and is also known as the *third eye* and the *brow chakra*. It is the seat of insight, intellect, and intuition.

The sixth energy tunnel fosters imagination, awareness of the subtle/energetic world, intuitive knowing, and inner vision. When you see something "with your mind's eye," you are seeing it with the sixth energy tunnel.

Someone with a clear, balanced, and developed brow tunnel usually has a keen intellect balanced with strong intuitive abilities. Such a person has a good imagination and can visualize things easily. A healthy sixth tunnel fosters the ability to grasp the big picture and expresses the prized but elusive faculty of intuition. The sixth tunnel is also associated with dreaming. Many people, including myself, believe that certain dreams can serve as premonitions. During the course of my life I have had hundreds of dreams that turned out to be premonitions. When these premonitions manifest in waking life I experience a déjà vu sensation. The sixth energy tunnel tunes us in to these exceptional experiences.

Have you ever had a peculiar feeling about a person, place, or event that you couldn't explain? Have you ever had a strange inkling that a certain event might take place, without any solid evidence to support it? These types of experiences are often called *gut feelings* or *intuitions*, and everybody has them. Unfortunately, many people tend to disregard their intuitions and gut feelings and choose instead to overrationalize their life situations. Well-known psychologist and researcher on consciousness Robert Ornstein points out, "Many intellectuals are to a certain extent afraid when intuition intrudes into their thought process; they are diffident and treat it gingerly; consciously or unconsciously they repress it."[7] Working with the sixth energy tunnel can greatly help to open up our repressed intuition and primal mind.

Physiologically, the indigo tunnel is located behind the center of the forehead or third eye, which is located a little above and between the eyebrows. It is associated with the pituitary gland, which is about the size of a pea and sits in a bony hollow called the *pituitary fossa,* behind the bridge of the nose and below the base of the brain, close to the optic nerves. The pituitary gland is considered the most important part of the endocrine system because it produces hormones that control the functions of the other endocrine glands:

Prolactin: Prolactin stimulates breast-milk production after childbirth. It also affects sex hormone levels from the ovaries in women and from the testes (testicles) in men, as well as fertility.

Growth hormone (GH): GH stimulates growth in childhood and is important for maintaining a healthy body composition and a sense of well-being in adults. In adults, GH is important for maintaining muscle mass and bone mass. It also affects fat distribution in the body.

Adrenocorticotropin hormone (ACTH): ACTH stimulates the production of cortisol by the adrenal glands. Cortisol, the so-called stress hormone, is vital to our survival. It helps maintain blood pressure and blood glucose (sugar) levels and is produced in larger amounts when we're under stress, especially after illness or injury.

Thyroid-stimulating hormone (TSH): TSH stimulates the thyroid gland to produce thyroid hormones, which regulate the body's metabolism, energy balance, growth, and nervous-system activity.

Luteinizing hormone (LH): LH stimulates testosterone production in men and egg release (ovulation) in women.

Follicle-stimulating hormone (FSH): FSH promotes sperm production in men and stimulates the ovaries to produce estrogen and develop eggs in women. LH and FSH work together to enable normal function of the ovaries and testes.

Antidiuretic hormone (ADH): ADH, also called *vasopressin,* regulates water balance in the body. It conserves body water by reducing the amount of water lost in urine.

Oxytocin: Oxytocin causes milk to flow from the breasts in breast-feeding women and may also help a woman in labor to progress.

Because it regulates so many processes of the body, it's no wonder the pituitary is considered the master gland.

+ Once you have your indigo-colored meditation fabric, board, or paper, get into a comfortable meditative AT position such as the yoga half-lotus. Simply sitting on the floor with your legs crossed is fine too; the main thing is to be in a comfortable position to view the color field in front of you.

+ Begin by closing your eyes, silently saying *I breathe me* just as in all the other AT sessions. After about two minutes of this passive breathing, open your eyes and hold your indigo drape in front of you close to the tip of your nose.

+ Focus on indigo with all your being. Internalize it while also concentrating on the area of your third eye, inside your forehead and above and a little higher than the center of your eyebrows. Breathe normally, and keep developing this meditative state for at least fifteen minutes or for however much time is comfortable for you to internalize indigo. If your arms feel tired, close your eyes, lay the drape in your lap, keep indigo in your mind, and after a minute or two, resume holding the drape.

+ Once you have fully internalized indigo, close your eyes and lay the drape in your lap.

+ With your eyes closed, keep the color indigo in your mind's eye.

+ Now place your hands on your forehead and perform AT using formulas related to the sixth energy tunnel. You can use just sixth tunnel formulas by silently repeating them, or mix them in with standard formulas. I prefer the latter. Some examples:

> *My pituitary gland is regulating my body perfectly.*
> *My body temperature is comfortable and stable.*
> *My metabolic rate is healthy for my body.*
> *My adrenaline is properly balanced, and I am ready for action.*
> *My energy distribution is even and vigorous.*
> *My heartbeat is calm and strong.*

+ Once you have finished with your physiological AT experience, perform psychological formulas by silently asking yourself simple questions related to the sixth energy tunnel and passively waiting for the answers. Use the above descriptions of the sixth tunnel and the color indigo to formulate your questions.

Some examples:

In what ways do I use my intellect in daily life?

In which specific events in my life have I used my intuition?

How strongly can I visualize with my mind's eye?

Am I able to stand back and see the big picture? If so, when I have done it?

Do I have the ability to perceive beyond what my eyes can see?

How do I use my deepest and most profound thoughts in my daily life?

Am I able to remember lucid dreams? What were they?

Do I experience premonitions during dreaming or while awake? Can I remember any of them?

✦ When you feel you are finished with your questions/answers, pick up your drape and hold it in front of you the same way as before, then open your eyes and focus on indigo until it is fully internalized once again. This could be almost immediately or might take a minute or two. Don't rush the process.

✦ End your session with an affirmation while staying "in the indigo" with eyes open. Say it out loud to the indigo and to your brow tunnel. Some examples:

My mind is clear and agile.

My imagination is vivid and powerful.

I am open to the intuition within me.

I can see the bigger picture of my life events and situations.

I am open to premonitions and gut feelings I may experience but also know they aren't always accurate.

I nurture profound insights and thoughts.

Training #23
Seventh Tunnel—Violet

Associated organ: brain

Associated gland: pineal

Associated problems: Some of the associated problems relating to the crown energy tunnel are depression, Parkinson's disease, schizophrenia, epilepsy, senile dementia, Alzheimer's, many mental disorders, confusion, dizziness, brain fog. Other problems include raised intracranial pressure resulting in headache, nausea, and vomiting; visual problems (since the pineal gland is very close to the pretectum), gait abnormalities, unsteadiness, diabetes insipidus, hypothalamic dysfunction.

Personality traits: balanced clear intention, spirituality, enjoyment of peaceful activities, clear sense of meaning in life, compassion, mental stability, lack of attachment to material possessions, general good health

Positive aspects of violet: reverence for all life, excellence in one's chosen profession, great mental powers, humanitarianism, pure idealism, egolessness, kindness, sense of justice, intuitiveness, faithfulness, sense of oneness

Negative aspects of violet: "superiority complex," lack of concern for and awareness of others, fanaticism, intolerance, dreaminess, tendency to judge others, inconsideration

---

The seventh tunnel is the highest and is located at the crown of the head or just slightly above; it is the avenue to higher states of consciousness. As we develop it, we become increasingly aware of consciousness itself, the eternal part of us that is beyond ego, thoughts, feelings, and body. This awareness can enhance harmony and peace in our lives. When fully stimulated, the crown tunnel fosters unity consciousness, the supramental understanding that separateness from anything, including what can't be seen (Creator, God, etc.), is but an illusion.

A person with a relatively clear, balanced, and developed crown tunnel is what might best be described as a spiritual (though not necessarily religious) person. Such a person usually spends regular time in prayer, meditation, or other devotions and enjoys peaceful activities. They have a sense of meaning in life and feel connected to a Higher Power or larger purpose. They may have glimpses of unity consciousness and spiritual bliss. They radiate goodwill and compassionate amusement at the twists and turns of life. They are mentally stable and fairly well grounded, and although they may be indifferent to many ordinary social conventions, they still maintain their bodies and at least a few relationships. Someone with a highly developed seventh tunnel is usually recognized as a spiritual teacher or master.

Physiologically, the seventh tunnel is associated with the pineal gland, regarded as one of the most important parts of the nervous system. The physiological functions of the pineal gland have been unknown by science until recent times; nevertheless, mystical traditions and esoteric schools have long known this area to be the connecting link between the physical and the spiritual worlds. Considered the most powerful and highest source of ethereal energy available to humans, the pineal gland is important in initiating supernatural powers. Development of psychic talents has also been closely associated with this tunnel of higher vision.

The pineal gland is located near the center of the brain between the two hemispheres, tucked in a groove where the two rounded thalamic bodies join. It's very close but a little higher up than the pituitary gland of the sixth energy tunnel. Unlike much of the rest of the brain, the pineal gland is not isolated from the body by the blood-brain barrier that separates the circulating blood from the brain extracellular fluid (BECF) in the central nervous system; in fact, it has profuse blood flow, second only to the kidneys. It is reddish gray, about the size of a pea (8 millimeters in humans), and is shaped like a pinecone, hence its name.

Melatonin, a derivative of the amino acid tryptophan, is produced by the pineal gland and is stimulated by darkness and inhibited by light. Photosensitive cells in the retina detect light and directly signal the suprachiasmatic nucleus (SCN), entraining its rhythm to the twenty-four-hour cycle in nature. The gland also helps the body convert signals from the nervous system to signals in the endocrine system, and in conjunction with the hypothalamus gland the pineal gland controls sex drive, hunger, thirst, and the biological clock that determines the body's normal aging process.

The major health risk to the pineal gland is calcification, which is a great cause for concern because it can happen at a very young age. In this process, the pineal gland accumulates calcium phosphate crystals, becomes hardened, and loses much of its functionality. There is a great deal of speculation as to what causes calcification of the pineal gland. Fluoride in water and toothpaste has been implicated in this process. In fact, many people believe that any food additives including artificial sweeteners may contribute to the problem. Although studies are not available to support the claim that the radiation from cell phones contributes to the pineal gland's calcification, that too has been implicated.

It is important to keep the pineal gland active because of the many important functions of this gland. When it is active, the pineal gland helps you to get good sleep; it also helps you to stay wide awake during the day. An active pineal gland will also ensure that neurological signals are clearly transmitted to the endocrine system, which includes the first energy tunnel (adrenals), the second tunnel (testes, ovaries), the third tunnel (pancreas), the fourth tunnel (thymus), the fifth tunnel (thyroid), and the sixth tunnel (pituitary). Without signals from the pineal gland, the other energy tunnels and their associated glands would not function.

Friends of mine who are naturopathic physicians (medical doctors who employ holistic and alternative treatments) have given me a short list of natural remedies that may help reduce pineal gland calcification:

Neem extract and oregano oil: These may help decalcify the pineal gland, purify other parts of the endocrine system, fortify the immune system, and act as a natural antibiotic in the body. For thousands of years in India, parts of the neem tree have been used to decalcify the pineal gland and open the third eye.

Raw apple cider vinegar: The malic acid in raw apple cider vinegar can be used to help detoxify your body, including the pineal gland. Be sure that the apple cider vinegar supplement you buy is raw and not processed. In addition to helping decalcify the pineal gland, raw apple cider vinegar can help your digestive system process foods better.

Essentials oils: Pure essential oils may help stimulate the pineal gland and decalcify it. Specifically, lavender, parsley, pine, sandalwood, pink lotus, and frankincense may be helpful in the decalcification process. Make sure the oils are pure and preferably single source; there is much contamination of essential oils by companies (many of them marketing their oil as "organic") that do not carefully source their oil. Essential oil enters the bloodstream through the skin in minute doses, such that a little bit of bad oil can result in its own set of problems. (A few companies with consistently high standards are Young Living, Floracopeia, and Dōterra.)

Melatonin: The pineal gland already produces the hormone melatonin, which affects the body's circadian rhythms of waking and sleeping. Melatonin is also associated with relaxation and visualization, and people often take melatonin supplements as a sleep aid or to help overcome jet lag due to travel. It is suggested that you always start with the smallest dosage possible and do not use any melatonin supplement for longer than three months.

Raw cacao: Raw, organic chocolate in its purest form can help detoxify the pineal gland because of cacao's high antioxidant content. Cacao also helps stimulate the third eye.

Iodine: Many of us have been exposed to sodium fluoride due to fluoridation of our water systems, and this has also resulted in the calcification of the pineal gland. Iodine, naturally occurring in plants such as seaweed, effectively improves the removal of sodium fluoride via urine. Unfortunately, the Western diet has left most of us deficient in this vital mineral. To avoid calcium deficiency when taking iodine supplements, a diet incorporating many organic foods such as kale, broccoli, almonds, oranges, flax seeds, sesame seeds, dill, thyme and other dried herbs is recommended. It is suggested that a non-GMO lecithin supplement is also taken to complement iodine intake.

Chlorophyll-rich superfoods: Supplements like spirulina, chlorella, wheatgrass, and blue-green algae are examples of chlorophyll-rich superfoods that offer similar benefits to eating leafy greens but with much more nutrition packed into a small serving. These supplements assist in the decalcification of the pineal gland due to their strong detoxification properties.

Other food remedies: In addition to the supplements listed above, there are many foods that help decalcify and improve the function of the pineal gland while detoxifying other parts of the body. These include cilantro, tamarind, goji berries, watermelon, bananas, honey, coconut oil, hemp seeds, seaweed, noni juice, garlic, chaga mushroom, and raw lemon juice.

+ Once you have your violet-colored meditation fabric, board, or paper, get into a comfortable meditative AT position such as the yoga half-lotus. Simply sitting on the floor with your legs crossed is fine too; the main thing is to be in a comfortable position to view the color field in front of you.

+ Begin by closing your eyes, silently saying *I breathe me* just as in all the other AT sessions. After about two minutes of this passive breathing, open your eyes and hold your violet drape in front of you close to the tip of your nose.

+ Focus on violet with all your being. Internalize it while also concentrating on the crown or top of your head. Breathe normally, and keep developing this meditative state for at least fifteen minutes or for however much time is comfortable for you to internalize violet. If your arms feel tired, close your eyes, lay the drape in your lap, keep violet in your mind, and after a minute or two resume holding the drape.

+ Once you have fully internalized violet, close your eyes and lay the drape in your lap.

+ With your eyes closed, keep the color violet in your mind's eye.

+ Now place your hands on the top of your head and perform AT using formulas related to the seventh energy tunnel. The seventh tunnel is special, as it is connected to our higher consciousness not only energetically but also physiologically, through signals sent via our nervous system. The AT formulas for this tunnel can be considered a review of all the previous energy tunnels, so they can include any or all of the formulas for the other six tunnels. If you need to, simply review the formulas for the other tunnels before beginning this exercise.

✦ Once you have finished with your physiological AT experience, perform psychological formulas by asking yourself simple questions related to the seventh energy tunnel, passively waiting for the answers. Use the above descriptions of the seventh tunnel and the color violet to formulate your silent questions. Some examples:

> *Do I feel a sense of balance in my life? If so, how? If not, what can change?*
> *Do I have a sense of meaning in my life? What is it?*
> *How do I experience spirituality?*
> *How well do I really know myself?*
> *How is my general health? What can I do to be healthier?*
> *What activities do I engage in that connect with the unity of nature and the cosmos?*

✦ When you feel finished with your questions/answers, pick up your drape and hold it in front of you the same way as before, then open your eyes and focus on violet until it is fully internalized once again. This could be almost immediately or might take a minute or two. Don't rush the process.

✦ End your session with an affirmation while staying "in the violet" with eyes open. Say it out loud to the indigo and to your brow tunnel. Some examples:

> *I am one with all creation.*
> *I am connected to vast inner wisdom.*
> *I consciously live my divine purpose.*
> *I am whole.*
> *I am beautiful.*
> *I am at peace.*
> *My energy resonates with divine light, acceptance, inspiration, and grace.*

For Western science the study of the chakras and acknowledgment of the etheric body is new and ongoing; yet the study and application of knowledge concerning the chakras by mystical traditions throughout the world have been continually and successfully practiced since roughly 1700 BCE.[8] For me, whether scientifically proven or not, effective techniques for personal growth rely on results. And the positive results of working with the seven energetic tunnels as described in this series of practices has been undeniable.

PART FOUR

༄

Techniques of Primal Mind, Autogenic Training, Our Senses, and the Natural World

10

Primal Connection with the
SENSE OF TOUCH

All of us know that we feel and experience our senses. But our modern culture of abstract language and exposure to all things electronic has in many ways disconnected us from our primal awareness of our ordinary physical and extraordinary nonphysical senses. And even though we may be peripherally aware of our natural senses, we don't honor them in the same way our primal ancestors did. We are educated to repress the full potential of our sensory self in order to live and function in modern technological society. Our education is almost always gleaned in indoor classrooms, and we graduate to work in such artificial environments. Many more examples could be cited here, but the bottom line is that our abstract language–training and indoors-oriented technological lifestyles too often replace our directly experiencing our natural human senses. As we proceed through the sensory trainings, this will become more apparent as we reconnect with some of the senses we don't normally attend to, and also reenergize some of our "normal" senses in novel ways.

As we become more aware of our senses, we tune into the fact that they are essential to human life, and by intentionally working with them on a psychophysiological level they can become a source of primal knowledge that can be used for personal growth and healing. In short, our senses can help us better connect to ourselves, others, and the entire matrix of the natural world of which we are part.

Most of us are born with healthy and intact senses that flourish unless they are somehow programmed, repressed, or deadened. Each of our senses is a beautiful, mysterious, *nonverbal* form of intelligence. Our language-based culture often thinks that by naming something, we actually know it. I can say I know this apple, but do I *really* know it? How about something more complex? Hey, there is a jet engine on that plane. I have a name for it, but do I really know it? Truth is, I haven't got a clue what it consists of and how it works except that it probably needs jet fuel.

With this in mind I'm going to introduce a helpful concept from Michael Cohen, a teacher of nature-based modalities and ecopsychologist specializing in reconnecting people with nature. Cohen points out that it is healthy for us to consider our senses as "nameless." In doing so we strip them of our preconceived word-based notions that trick us into thinking we know something because we have a name for it. This allows us to experience things as they truly are, through our senses. Our senses consist of what Cohen calls *attraction relationships,* not words. For example, through our senses we are attracted to the smell of a fragrant flower, the sound of the ocean, the soft coat of a cute puppy, a gorgeous sunset. Our senses attract us to the whole of the natural world and its ways, including the inner nature of other people. Each natural attraction we feel means one or more of our natural senses have awakened and their energies have brought them into our field of consciousness. In his programs Cohen uses an acronym to remember the four qualities of our senses: NIAL.

Namelessness: nonlanguage ways of relating, knowing, and feeling

Intelligence: the natural ability for attractions to blend in supportive ways

Attractions: natural energies that draw things together

Love: our ability to enjoyably feel nature's attraction process

Cohen says, "When we think in ways that exclude NIAL, we end up with stories and relationships that continuously conflict each other.

These stories often lead us to a stressed state of being. Without NIAL, we think our way into destructive perceptions and problems of race, nationality, sex, religion, and economics."[1] Cohen also believes (as do I) that we have become estranged from many of our senses by living most of our lives indoors. This has led us to DE-NIAL!

I'm going to assume that everyone reading this is familiar with our five ordinary senses that we have been educated about since grade school, and that were first elucidated by Aristotle around 350 BCE: sight (ophthalmoception), hearing (audioception), taste (gustaoception), smell (olfacoception), and touch (tactioception). A broadly accepted definition of a sense comes from *Webster's*: "one of the five natural powers (touch, taste, smell, sight, and hearing) through which you receive information about the world around you." There is no firm agreement as to the number of senses we have because of differing definitions of what constitutes a sense. Scientifically, the senses are frequently divided into interoceptive and exteroceptive. Interoceptive senses are senses that perceive sensations in internal organs. Exteroceptive senses are those that perceive the body's own position, motion, and state, which are further known as *proprioceptive senses*. These external senses include the traditional five (sight, hearing, touch, smell, and taste), as well as thermoception (sensing temperature differences) and magnetoception (sensing direction). Proprioceptive senses also include nociception (sensing pain), equilibrioception (sensing balance), proprioception (a sense of the position and movement of the parts of one's own body).

We now have extensive research on other types of senses and perception that are called variously *nontraditional senses, nontraditional internal senses* (we experience many of these in our AT), and *perception not based on a specific sensory organ* (also experienced during AT). There are many lists of senses (in addition to the ordinary five) that have been formulated by researchers, scientists, and the medical community, among others. Some of these lists have only a few additions to the traditional five, while others have many. In my research the most compressive work on human senses and sensitivities, especially with regard to our AT and PM work, has been compiled through experiential exploration by Michael Cohen. The following list is reprinted here with his permission. Please take a few moments to review it before we move on. I have found it very enlightening.

THE 54 NATURAL SENSES AND SENSITIVITIES
The Radiation Senses

1. Sense of light and sight, including polarized light
2. Sense of seeing without eyes, such as heliotropism or the sun sensing of plants
3. Sense of color
4. Sense of moods and identities attached to colors
5. Sense of awareness of one's own visibility or invisibility and consequent camouflaging
6. Sensitivity to radiation other than visible light, including radio waves, X-rays, etc.
7. Sense of temperature and temperature change
8. Sense of season, including ability to insulate, hibernate, and winter sleep
9. Electromagnetic sense and polarity, which includes the ability to generate current (as in the nervous system and brain waves) or other energies

The Feeling Senses

10. Hearing, including resonance, vibrations, sonar and ultrasonic frequencies
11. Awareness of pressure, particularly underground, underwater, and to wind and air
12. Sensitivity to gravity
13. The sense of excretion for waste elimination and protection from enemies
14. Feeling, particularly touch on the skin

15. Sense of weight, gravity, and balance
16. Space or proximity sense
17. Coriolus sense, or awareness of effects of Earth's rotation
18. Sense of motion, body movement sensations, and sense of mobility

The Chemical Senses

19. Smell with and beyond the nose
20. Taste with and beyond the tongue
21. Appetite or hunger for food, water, and air
22. Hunting, killing, or food-obtaining urges
23. Humidity sense, including thirst, evaporation control, and the acumen to find water or evade a flood
24. Hormonal sense, as to pheromones and other chemical stimuli

The Mental Senses

25. Pain, external and internal (numbers 25 through 27 are attractions to seek additional natural attractions in order to support and strengthen well-being, or attractions to run for your life)
26. Mental or spiritual distress
27. Sense of fear, dread of injury, death, or attack.
28. Procreative urges, including sexual awareness, courting, love, mating, paternity or maternity, and raising offspring
29. Sense of play, sport, humor, pleasure, and laughter
30. Sense of physical place, navigation senses, including detailed awareness of land and seascapes, of the positions of the sun, moon, and stars
31. Sense of time and rhythm
32. Sense of electromagnetic fields
33. Sense of weather changes
34. Sense of emotional place, of community, belonging, support, trust, and thankfulness
35. Sense of self, including friendship, companionship, and power

36. Domineering and territorial sense

37. Colonizing sense, including compassion and receptive awareness of one's fellow creatures, sometimes to the degree of being absorbed into a superorganism

38. Horticultural sense and the ability to cultivate crops as is done by ants that grow fungus, by fungus that farm algae, or birds that leave food to attract their prey

39. Language and articulation sense used to express feelings and convey information in every medium, from the bees' dance to human literature

40. Sense of humility, appreciation, ethics

41. Senses of form and design

42. Sense of reason, including memory and the capacity for logic and science

43. Sense of mind and consciousness

44. Intuition or subconscious deduction

45. Aesthetic sense, including creativity and appreciation of beauty, music, literature, form, design, and drama

46. Psychic capacity, such as foreknowledge, clairvoyance, clairaudience, psychokinesis, astral projection, and possibly certain animal instincts and plant sensitivities

47. Sense of biological and astral time, awareness of past, present, and future events

48. The capacity to hypnotize other creatures

49. Relaxation and sleep, including dreaming, meditation, brainwave awareness

50. Sense of pupation, including cocoon building and metamorphosis

51. Sense of excessive stress and capitulation

52. Sense of survival by joining a more established organism

53. Spiritual sense, including conscience, capacity for sublime love, ecstasy, a sense of sin, profound sorrow, and sacrifice

54. Sense of unity, of natural attraction aliveness as the singular essence/spirit and source of all our other senses

Working with even a portion of this list is beyond the scope of this book. Plus, we have plenty of opportunities to learn about, awaken, and reawaken our primary senses that have become stagnant or atrophied. So in this chapter I'm focusing on the primal awareness of touch, sight, hearing, and smell. Most of these trainings will have nature as a component in one way or the other. I'm not introducing trainings for our fifth primary sense, that of taste. This is mostly because 80 percent of taste is actually smell.

INTEGRATING PM TECHNIQUES INTO THE PRACTICE

Autogenic training is a wonderful and enlightening tool with many applications for increased physical and psychological wellness based primarily on techniques that alter our physiology. By adding affirmations, visualizations, and meditations of our energy tunnels to these physiological techniques we take the standard autogenic training techniques further into the realm of holistic healing and enlightenment.

However, to make our work with autogenic training truly holistic we must also include the natural world of which we will always be a part. Deep connection to the natural world is a significant portion of what I am calling primal mind (PM). Spontaneous primal experiences in nature can be awesome. Learning from a nature guide or experienced naturalist can be extremely enlightening. These experiences touch our primal mind in significant ways.

The goal of the second half of this book is to add autogenic training techniques into intentionally created primal mind experiences so that we take AT and PM into realms of self-discovery, healing, and altered states of consciousness that are truly holistic. By integrating AT into PM experiences of awakening our senses and immersing our entire organism in the natural world we open ourselves to holistic altered states of consciousness that far surpass what is experienced when AT and PM are experienced separately.

Throughout the rest of the book I will provide examples of how to integrate AT into the PM techniques that follow. But now that you are familiar with AT and know what works for you, you can decide at any moment what AT formulas to inject into the AT-PM trainings. You will also learn to integrate PM formulas. As the AT formulas aid us in creating a deeper connection to our inner selves, the PM formulas will allow us to draw the connection between that inner self and nature. You will see examples of some PM formulas throughout the following exercises, but feel free to create your own formulas that resonate with your engagement in the exercise in that particular time and place in nature. Although I provide the guidelines and suggestions that have been proven effective, the AT-PM trainings are much more free-form. Even though some of these trainings are intentionally designed to push your limits my suggestion is to embrace them with a light and joyful heart and enjoy yourself!

THE SENSE OF TOUCH

I'm going to begin our primal-mind training with a sense that we are intimately familiar with, that of touch. I'm choosing this one first because it is the only one of the five ordinary senses that we can't easily turn off. You can close your eyes and imagine what it's like to be blind, and you can stop up your ears and get some idea as to what it's like to be deaf. You can hold your nose or close your mouth. While your other four senses (sight, hearing, smell, and taste) are located in specific parts of the body, your sense of touch is found all over. This is because the sense of touch originates in the bottom layer of the skin, called the *dermis*. The dermis is filled with many tiny nerve endings that give you information about the things that your body comes in contact with. They do this by carrying the information to the spinal cord, which sends messages to the brain where the feeling is registered. This is the part of the somatic sensory system that is responsible for the sense of touch (see table 10.1, page 130, for more

TABLE 10.1. THE SENSORY MODALITIES REPRESENTED BY THE SOMATOSENSORY SYSTEMS

Modality	Submodality	Sub-submodality	Somatosensory pathway (body)	Somatosensory pathway (face)
Pain	sharp cutting pain	none	neospinothalamic	spinal trigeminal
	dull burning pain	none	paleospinothalamic	
	deep aching pain	none	archispinothalamic	
Temperature	warm/hot	none	paleospinothalamic	
	cool/cold	none	neospinothalamic	
	itch/tickle & crude touch	none	paleospinothalamic	
Touch	discriminative touch	touch	medial lemniscal	main sensory trigeminal
		pressure		
		flutter		
		vibration		
Proprioception	position: static forces	muscle length		
		muscle tension		
		joint pressure		
	movement: dynamic forces	muscle length		
		muscle tension		
		joint pressure		
		joint angle		

on sensory modalities). As we saw in figure 1.1 (page 7), the peripheral nervous system has two parts. The autonomic nervous system is the one related to AT (internal). The somatic sensory nervous system is its counterpart (external). This system has nerve receptors that help you feel when something comes into contact with your skin, such as when a person or anything else brushes up against you or when you intentionally touch something. These sensory receptors are generally known as *touch receptors* and *pressure receptors*. You also have nerve receptors that feel pain and temperature changes such as hot and cold.

Fine touch (or discriminative touch) is a sensory modality that allows you to sense and localize touch. The form of touch in which localization is not possible is known as *crude touch*. The posterior column–medial lemniscus pathway is the pathway responsible for the sending of fine-touch information to the cerebral cortex. Crude touch (or nondiscriminative touch) is a sensory modality that allows you to sense that something has touched you, without being able to localize where you were touched (as opposed to fine touch). Its fibers are carried in the spinothalamic tract, unlike fine touch, which is carried in the dorsal column. As fine touch normally works parallel with crude touch, you will be able to localize touch until fibers carrying fine touch have been disrupted. Then you will feel the touch but will be unable to identify where you were touched.

Before we move on, here are some not-so-well-known facts about our incredible sense of touch:

Different parts of our body have more or fewer touch receptors. This is something you will discover in training #24. Certain parts like the face, lips, tongue, and fingers have lots when compared to the small of your back, your chest, and your thighs.

You have a special system for feeling emotional and social touch. We basically have two systems of touch. The system we used in the two previous trainings is called *discriminative touch,* and it's the one that "gives us the facts." But then there's the emotional touch system. This is not just a different kind of information that's conveyed by the same sensors in the skin that allow you to feel a stick or a tree or cold water. It's a completely different set of sensors and nerve fibers that wind up in a different part of your brain and are mediated by special sensors called *C tactile fibers,* which convey information much more slowly. It's more vague in terms of where the touch is happening, but it sends information to a part of the brain called the *posterior insula* that is crucial for social-bonding touch. This includes things like a hug from a friend, the touch you got as a child from your mother, and also romantic/sexual touch.

You have a special system that makes pain hurt. Again, we have two systems for this. The first has sensors that tell you exactly where the pain is, how strong it is, etc. And then there's another system that just conveys the negative emotional aspect of the pain.

Your sense of touch gets worse as you age. First, areas of the touch-sensing parts of your brain that you use a lot tend to expand and take over areas not used as much. For example, a right-handed baseball pitcher uses his right hand way more often than his left, resulting in the area of his brain that processes information from his right hand to expand. Also, we all lose touch receptors over the course of our lives. It's not like we have them until a certain age, then they suddenly disappear; we lose them very, very slowly. They peak around age sixteen or eighteen, then begin to disappear slowly. We also lose pain and temperature receptors, which might actually be a good thing. It may be that when you're older you might not feel as much surface pain on your skin. But there are other notable implications of this: it may be that part of the reason it becomes harder to achieve orgasm as you grow older is that touch receptors in the skin of the genitals become less dense. This is also one of the factors that lead the elderly to take falls. We stay upright in part because of sensations on the bottom of our feet, and we get less of that information the older we get.

Touch is crucial for a baby's development. Kids raised throughout the world in orphanages from the time they were babies, and also babies in other situations where they barely get touched, have a host of emotional problems, including depression and high instances of schizophrenia, bipolar disorder, and other issues. And they also have a whole raft of physical ailments, such as weakened immune systems, and skin ailments. This is why, nowadays, when premature infants are born and put in incubators, they're taken out for a few hours a day and pressed against a parent's (usually mother's) skin. Initially, when incubators were first invented, people thought you should just leave the baby in there alone so he wouldn't get infected. But then they might not get touched for the first two months of life, which turns out to be disastrous.

Training #24
Primal Touch Sensitivity

Along with two forms of touch mentioned earlier, fine touch and crude touch, we also have areas of our body that are more or less sensitive to touch. Here is an insightful training technique:

+ For this technique you'll need to have a partner. Aside from a partner you'll need a ruler that measures in millimeters, two toothpicks, a sheet of paper, and something to write with.
+ Don't tell your partner what you are going to do yet. If he or she is curious just say you are doing a little experiment that won't take long and won't hurt. If you are using paper, first copy table 10.2 on page 135 (or you can just write the results in the table provided).
+ When ready, have your partner close her eyes, and explain that you are going to gently poke her with either one or two toothpicks on various places on her skin. Her job is to tell you whether or not she feels one poke or two pokes. To make sure she is not cheating, she needs to either wear a blindfold or keep her eyes closed.
+ Without telling your partner this, hold the two toothpicks so that the points

measure 1 mm apart and lightly poke her on the palm of her hand. Ask her if she felt one or two pricks on her skin. If she says one, separate the two points of the toothpicks so that they measure 2 mm apart and lightly poke her in the palm again. Keep pulling the points apart (refer to the chart) until she says that she feels two points. Record the measurement at which she felt two points on the palm of her hand.

+ Repeat this step with the other parts of the body listed on the chart. (Other areas you could try are the back of a finger, back of the hand, wrist, neck, stomach, top of the foot, sole of the foot, calf, thigh, forehead, nose, lip, and ear.) Record the smallest distance at which each area of the body felt two distinct points when poked with the toothpicks. Now have your partner try the same thing on you.

What just happened?

The ability to distinguish between one point or two points of sensation depends on how dense the mechanoreceptors are in the area of the skin being touched. You both most likely found which areas of the body are much more sensitive to touch than other areas. Highly sensitive areas such as the fingertips and tongue can have as many as 100 pressure receptors in one cubic centimeter. Less sensitive areas, such as the back, can have as few as ten pressure receptors in one cubic centimeter. Because of this, areas such as your back are much less responsive to touch and can gather less information about what is touching them than your fingertips can.

Next is a training technique you can do outside in nature by yourself.

Training #25
Touching Nature with Your Hands and Subtle Body

+ Grab a pencil or marker and go outside anywhere there are trees; tell the place you are there to learn.
+ Collect (from the ground) six similar-size sticks (both in diameter and length). Break the length if needed to make them all the same length.

TABLE 10.2. PRIMAL TOUCH RESULTS

	1 mm	2 mm	3 mm	4 mm	5 mm	10 mm	20 mm
Palm of hand							
Tip of finger							
Upper arm							
Back							
Cheek							

+ Sit down, close your eyes, and place the sticks in front of you.

+ Complete an AT-PM session using any standard AT formulas you choose while performing PM formulas between the standard formulas like we have done before. Examples of PM formulas to say to yourself include *My hands have incredible abilities of perception; I can touch, feel, and remember anything I hold; I can touch with my fingers at the most minute and fine levels; I don't need my sight to see what I am touching.*

+ With eyes still closed, pick up one stick from your pile and mark it with your pencil or marker. Then take your time and familiarize yourself intimately with your stick—its shape, texture, any special qualities like bumps or ridges. Take your time, and try to internalize and remember everything about that stick. Use your experience with visualization to visualize the stick as well.

+ When you are ready, still with your eyes closed, return your stick to the pile and mix them up.

+ Do at least one AT and one PM formula. Don't skip this part because performing your formulas will help you find your stick, and furthermore, your stick might still be holding some of your body heat.

+ After silently saying the formulas, breathe normally and visualize your stick for a few moments. With eyes still closed, pick up the sticks one at a time and examine each of them with your fingers until you find the one you think you marked.

+ Open your eyes, and see if you have found the correct stick.

What conclusions about your sense of touch can you draw from this exercise? I like doing this training with rocks too. Other natural items you could include in this exercise are pinecones, fruit (apples, berries, etc.), and acorns, all of which can be amazingly similar while also being unique. Sometimes in my groups we do a variation on this PM exercise in the forest. For this you'll need a partner:

+ Shut or blindfold your eyes.

+ Without speaking, have your partner guide you to a tree in the area that is fairly similar to others close by. Then, in a similar way as previously with the sticks, get to know the tree by your sense of touch, by your feelings, and through visualization. Take as much time as you need to fully internalize this magnificent living entity.

✦ When you feel ready, have your partner guide you away from your tree just far enough so that you don't exactly know where it is.

✦ Now open your eyes and go back and try to find your tree. Please don't turn into a tracker by trying to find footprints; that's not part of this exercise. Go from tree to tree until you find yours, or not. If you're not sure, your partner can tell you, but in most cases I have seen that when someone finds her tree there is no doubt.

This can be a fun PM activity for kids too. When working with youngsters I usually guide them to a tree that's a little different, maybe bigger or smaller or with fewer or more leaves and branches, until they get the hang of it.

Training #26
Touch the Earth—Barefoot Walking in Nature

This training has evolved throughout the years from my 2002 book on walking techniques, *Earthwalks for Body and Spirit: Exercises to Restore Our Sacred Bond with the Earth.* For those of you familiar with that book I invite you to try this version of a walk that adds an AT component, which was not included in my earlier book. AT brings an even deeper level of primal mind to an already powerful experience of touch.

Taking your shoes off instantly changes your view of the world. Your personality transforms, you relax and let down your guard, and suddenly you feel not so insulated from the world. The soles of our feet are wonderful sensory organs that we tend to keep wrapped up and suffocated, but when they are freed to the air and the earth, the sun and the water, they can provide us with untold amounts of pleasure and discovery as we explore the world of walking in nature in a new and fascinating way. The physical sensation of feeling earth, moss, grass, leaves, water, rocks, mud, wood, and a myriad of other textures and surfaces creates a whole new world at the feeling level when we walk on the bare soles of our feet. But this is much more than a purely physical experience; this is also a state of mind. Taking off your shoes to walk the earth is an expression of your desire to be close to your mother, to really feel her, to shed the artificiality of the technological world and walk the same as the rest of her nonhuman children. Only humans insulate themselves from the earth as we do. This technique of primal touching is an invitation for you to let your feet escape their bondage and run free.

Since most of us are not accustomed to walking outdoors without shoes let's review some simple points before starting. The first is common sense. If you really pay attention to what you're doing, walking barefoot is not dangerous in the least. I know people who never wear shoes, ever, and they are perfectly happy. In fact, they would have it no other way. So the first thing to do is let your perception of the world open up a little to include the fact that shoes aren't absolutely necessary for survival. Now add to that the fact that the soles of your feet are highly sensitive and will need to be cared for with love and gentleness until they become familiar with the world again. My suggestion is to care for your bare feet as you would for a small child who has just learned to walk. You wouldn't take a small child for a five-mile hike in the desert, or let him run into the street or climb on high rocks. Neither should you do these things barefoot until you are ready. So start off like a child learning to walk; walk in the soft grass, in your yard, or go to a park or nature center where they have manicured trails for walking. Try exploring all kinds of different walking surfaces while being extremely gentle and careful. And above all, enjoy!

The following is an AT session specifically designed for this training. But of course feel free to modify it:

+ Find a place outdoors where you will be comfortable walking barefoot. If you are superattentive you can actually walk barefoot anywhere; just be mindful.

+ Once you have arrived at your destination and are comfortable, take off your shoes and begin your AT. I suggest you either lie flat on your back or sit on the ground with your back against a tree; if you're in a park with benches, sit there using a meditative position.

+ Engage in two minutes of passive breathing, slowly repeating *I breathe me.*

+ Passively focus on each of the areas below, one at a time.

+ Starting with your dominant arm, silently repeat three times *My right* (or *left*) *arm is heavy.*

+ Silently repeat three times *My heartbeat is calm and strong.*

+ Silently repeat six times *The earth awaits my feet.*

+ Silently repeat three times *My solar plexus is warm.*

+ Silently repeat three times *My legs and feet are warm.*

+ Silently repeat six times *My feet are sensitive and receptive.*

+ While still aware of the warmth in your legs and feet and how magnificently sensitive your feet are, say to yourself *I am very quiet.*

+ Remain relaxed for a minute or two.

+ Cancel.

+ Repeat this sequence two more times.

+ After your final cancel, begin walking in a very aware manner, in which you "place" your feet, attentive to exactly where you want them to go as you walk. Avoid shuffling or dragging your feet. Pay extremely close attention to what is on the ground in front of you as you walk. If you see something interesting on either side of you, then stop to look at it; don't walk while looking to the side because then you are not watching where you are placing your feet.

+ Breathe deeply and relax while remaining attentive. Walk slowly, and feel the new sensations; they are just that, new sensations. It is not uncommon for the first few minutes of barefoot walking in nature to be an experience of sensory overload. The pure volume of new sensations can bring on strong primal feelings of love for nature and for yourself as part of nature, and possibly regret for not having done this sooner. It's okay, you're doing it now, and now is what matters. Connect to the primal-mind awareness that our ancient ancestors experienced walking this way all the time. Walk slowly, and if you need to, cry; or if you yearn to laugh and jump up and down, then do it. There are no rules here, especially without shoes. I suggest slowly walking barefoot for at least an hour. In my workshops we usually spend half a day enjoying this experience.

✦ As you get used to the feeling of walking barefoot, challenge yourself to explore many different types of terrains. Walking in puddles or on pine needles, soft cool earth, dry rocky earth, leaves, stone, wood, etc.—each has a unique feeling and energy. The sensations you can experience are as diverse as nature herself. Open yourself up, walk the earth with your bare bottoms, and you will never be the same again . . .

It is my hope that you resonated with this training to the point that you will keep on doing it in the future. By taking short barefoot walks two or three times a week, you will probably feel comfortable walking two or three miles after a month or so. It is always a good idea to carry shoes in a backpack and bring them with you just in case your feet do get sore as you progress to more challenging terrain. If you have the habit of finding your mind wandering while you walk, then it might also be a good idea to put Band-Aids and disinfectant in the pack along with your shoes. When I first started walking barefoot for extended periods and wanted to really get out in the wilderness I would often (and still do) walk or hike with shoes or boots on until I got to a location where I wanted to walk barefoot. This is a safe and effective way to explore diverse types of terrain.

Barefoot walking is a great activity to do with friends. Sharing the experience and the sensations can sometimes add even more to the feelings of discovery, but I have also enjoyed many moments walking barefoot alone in the middle of a wilderness, at a dead slow speed, soaking up every feeling and sensation, with every part of each foot, with every step. Anyway you look at it, barefoot walking on the earth is like coming home to your true primal mother.

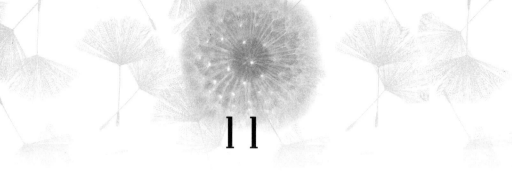

11

Primal Connection with the
SENSES OF SIGHT AND HEARING

We usually think of vision in terms of visual acuity, like when we get our eyes tested for the ability to clearly see letters on a chart. That of course is an important part of vision, but it's not everything. Vision is the process of deriving meaning from what is seen. It is a complex learned and developed set of functions that involve a multitude of skills. About 80 percent of what we learn from the world around us is due to perception, learning, cognition, and activities that are mediated through vision.

THE PHYSIOLOGY OF SIGHT

The ultimate purpose of vision is to act on what we see and respond to that either with our muscles or through cognitive response (understanding). The process of vision can be broken down into three general categories: (1) visual acuity and visual field; (2) visual motor abilities; and (3) visual perception. *Visual acuity* refers to clarity of sight. It is commonly measured using the Snellen eye chart that notes, for example, vision that is 20/20, 20/50, or 20/200. Our visual field is the complete central and peripheral range, or panorama of vision. *Visual motor ability* refers to alignment. Alignment has to do with eye posture. If the eyes are straight and aligned, the eye posture is termed *phoric*. If an eye turns in, out, up, or down compared to the other eye, then the eyes are not straight or aligned and the condition is termed *strabismus*. Exotropia is a form of strabismus wherein an eye turns out, esotropia is where an eye turns in, hypertropia is when an eye turns up, and hypotropia is when an eye turns down. These can also occur in combination, such as hyper-exotropia, or hypo-esotropia.

The ways in which we look are as follows:

- **Fixation:** the ability to steadily and accurately gaze at an object of regard
- **Pursuit:** the ability to smoothly and accurately track or follow a moving object
- **Saccades:** the ability to quickly and accurately look or scan from one object to another
- **Accommodation:** the ability to accurately focus on an object of regard, sustain that focusing of the eyes, and to change focusing when looking at different distances
- **Convergence:** the ability to accurately aim the eyes at an object of regard and to track an object as it moves toward and away from us
- **Binocularity:** the integration of accommodation and convergence
- **Stereopsis:** depth perception

The way in which we visually perceive are as follows:

- **Visual-motor integration:** eye-hand, eye-foot, and eye-body coordination
- **Visual-auditory integration:** the ability to relate and associate what is seen and heard
- **Visual memory:** the ability to remember and recall information that is seen
- **Visual closure:** the ability to fill in the gaps; i.e., to complete a visual picture based on seeing only some of the parts

- **Spatial relationships:** the ability to know where I am in relation to objects and space around me and to know where objects are in relation to one another
- **Figure-ground discrimination:** the ability to discern form and object from background

Most of us know or have heard the basic terms used for parts of the eye. But let's just take a quick look at this amazing feature of the human body. Your eye is about 2.5 centimeters in length and weighs about 7 grams. Light passes through the cornea, pupil, and lens before hitting the retina. The iris is a muscle that controls the size of the pupil and therefore the amount of light that enters the eye. Also, the color of your eyes is determined by the iris. By the way, the color of your eyes has nothing to do with how well you can see or perceive.

The vitreous or vitreous humor is a clear gel that provides constant pressure to maintain the shape of the eye. The retina is the area of the eye that contains the receptors (rods and cones) that respond to light. The receptors respond to light by generating electrical impulses that travel out of the eye through the optic nerve to the brain.

Six bands of muscles attach to the eyeball to control the ability of the eye to look up and down and side to side. These muscles are controlled by three cranial nerves. Four of the muscles are controlled by the oculomotor nerve, one muscle is controlled by the trochlear nerve and one muscle is controlled by the abducens nerve.

The retina is the back part of the eye that contains the cells that respond to light. These specialized cells are called *photoreceptors*. There are two types: rods and cones. The rods are most sensitive to light and dark changes and shape and movement and contain only one type of light-sensitive pigment. Rods are not good for color vision. In a dim room, we use mainly our rods; otherwise we are color blind. Rods are more numerous than cones in the periphery of the retina. Next time you want to see a dim star at night, try to look at it with your peripheral vision and use this "rod vision" to see the dim star. There are about 120 million rods in the human retina.

The cones are not as sensitive to light as the rods. However, cones are sensitive to one of three different colors: green, red, and blue. Signals from the cones are sent to the brain, which then translates these messages into the perception of color. Cones, however, work only in bright light. That's why you can't see color very well in dark places. So the cones are used for color vision and are better suited for detecting fine details. There are about six million cones in the human retina. Some people can't tell some colors from others, what is referred to as *color blindness*. Someone who is color blind does not have a particular type of cone in the retina, or one type of cone may be weak. In the general population, about 8 percent of all men are color blind, while only about 0.5 percent of all women are color blind.

The fovea is the central region of the retina that provides for the clearest vision. In the fovea there are no rods, only cones. The cones are also packed closer together in the fovea than in the rest of the retina. Also, blood vessels and nerve fibers go around the fovea so light has a direct path to the photoreceptors.

Here is an easy way to demonstrate the sensitivity of your foveal vision. Stare at the *g* in the word *light* in the middle of the following sentence:

Your vision is best when light falls on the fovea.

The *g* in *light* will be clear, but words on either side of the word *light* will not be clear or as clear. Notably, one part of the retina does not contain any photoreceptors. This is called the *blind spot,* meaning any image that falls on this region will not be seen. It is in this region that the optic nerves come together and exit the eye on their way to the brain.

To find your blind spot, look at the image below or draw it on a piece of paper:

●   ✚

Close your left eye.

Hold this image about twelve inches away. With your right eye, look at the dot. Slowly bring the image (or move your head) slightly closer or farther away while looking at the dot. At a certain distance, the + will disappear from sight. This is when the + falls on the blind spot of your retina. Reverse the process. Close your right eye and look at the + with your left eye. Move the image slowly closer or farther away and the dot should disappear.

There are many tests, games, and activities out there to learn more about our vision, but here we are most interested in primal vision, so below are two of my favorite trainings. Although space doesn't allow us to go into an in-depth treatment of sense of hearing, both of these trainings include hearing as a major component.

Training #27
Experiencing Sight, Sound, and Rhythm with Heightened Awareness

I'm going to explain the following techniques from the primal point of view of being in a forest, up in a tree. If you don't feel comfortable with my suggestion of going up a tree you can engage these techniques from the ground. Simply disregard the part about going up and staying in the tree. But I highly recommend you do your best to get up in a tree in the way I'm going to describe. This technique takes some effort, but it is so powerful in terms of primal awareness that it is well worth the effort. In any case, the idea here is to get yourself out of the straight-lined urban grid and into a natural environment such as a forest, and then for those who choose to, to get up off the ground and into a tree to be able to look out and over a natural area in a way that you feel safe and comfortable enough to remain in the tree for a number of hours. Although this can be accomplished in a number of ways I'm going to outline my preferred way, not only because it is a safe practice but also because it allows you to be very still and comfortable, which is really important in order to inspire you to keep practicing.

The ideal way to do this practice (but sometimes we just have to work with what we have available) is to climb about eight feet up a medium-size straight-trunk tree located on a gently sloping hill in a forest lying at a distance from the hustle and bustle of the modern world. I try to find a tree in an inspiring location that is approximately twelve to eighteen inches in diameter and is relatively free of branches from six to eight feet above the ground. I don't really want or need lower branches because I'm going to sit in the tree by anchoring a tree stand to the tree. (If you already have a tree stand and know how to use it, you can skip the next three paragraphs.)

A tree stand is a piece of equipment that you can find at any sporting goods shop that caters to hunters (hunters use them to stay hidden from prey), or you can buy them online. If you go the online route I suggest you go to a sporting goods shop first and check them out to familiarize yourself with them in person. The tree stand is a small lightweight platform that folds up for carrying and unfolds for placing onto a tree trunk by way of a heavy-duty strap-and-locking mechanism. When properly installed, this type of platform is completely harmless to the tree. Never buy a tree stand that uses a chain or bolts to attach to the tree; always use the strap-on type, and I recommend a lightweight model unless you are a very heavy person. Tree stands come in a wide variety of configurations, from super simple to elaborate and expensive. I prefer the simple kind. In any case, follow the manufacturer's recommendation as to which tree stand is best for you. Most salespeople who sell tree stands use them themselves and are quite knowledgeable.

The tree-stand platform straps to the tree and then locks into place when you unfold it, creating a platform for your feet and a seat for you to sit on. Once you have the tree stand in place and you are up in it, you can secure yourself with a safety strap* so that you now have a very comfortable, safe, and unique way to submerge yourself in the magic of the

---

*Some tree stands come with an integrated safety bar. The simple kinds don't, so a safety strap or rope is necessary. Safety straps are easy to use and full instructions on use, are included.

forest. To get to the proper height I usually use either a lightweight ladder or strap-on steps that can be purchased with the tree stand. There are also "climbing" tree-stand stands, but these take a lot of strength to use. Strap-on steps are great, especially if you have a private wooded area that you can return to frequently so that you can leave the steps attached to the tree for periods of time. If you are not completely comfortable doing this the first time you can ask a friend to join you for safety.

Please make sure to prepare properly before using the tree stand. You must familiarize yourself completely with how to anchor the steps (or ladder) and tree stand to the tree before you go up. I suggest practicing the anchoring of the tree stand at waist level, and then sitting and standing on it, and climbing on and off it many times before going up any higher. Also, familiarize yourself with and *always* use the safety strap. Commercially available tree stands are well built and very safe once you get the feel of them, and once you are comfortable with your tree stand it will become like a good friend. I have used tree stands for over twenty years of hunting deer (I don't hunt anymore) and for this AT-PM technique for many more years. In fact, they make possible such a wide range of enlightening experiences that using them can become quite addictive.

Whether you are in a tree or on the ground, the first thing to do is to take some deep breaths, relax, and settle in. Try to become as still as the tree trunk. In the first moments it's not important to do anything special except for simply getting yourself comfortable and quiet. This will be happening both internally as you become relaxed and externally as your local environment relaxes to your being there. After you practice with the tree stand a few times you'll begin to recognize the brief transition time between your entrance into the forest and the corresponding intrusion felt by the beings that live there (which feels like everything is holding its breath). After you become quiet the forest will return to its normal activity. When this transition time has passed, you now have open to you myriad opportunities for discovery in the realm of perception and experience. Here is a sample sequence that you can alter as you gain experience.

For this technique we will be combining standard AT formulas with PM formulas relating to depth perception, expanding our senses, seeing the forest in new ways, and engaging with the flow of the forest. During the course of these experiences you can use all the standard formulas or just the ones that are most effective for you. During the PM formulas (between the standard formulas) we will open our eyes to engage the forest visually. Of course, during the standard formulas our eyes are closed.

+ As always, engage in at least two minutes passive breathing, silently repeating *I breathe me.*

+ Passively focus on each of the areas below, one at a time.

+ Starting with your dominant arm, silently repeat three times *My right* (or *left*) *arm is heavy.* Silently repeat three times *I can see into the forest deeply.* Now open your eyes and gaze as far as you can into the forest and focus your vision way out in front of you. Passively open yourself to the depth of the forest for a few minutes, then close your eyes.

+ Silently repeat three times *My arms and legs are heavy and warm.*

+ Silently repeat three times *I clearly see my place in this forest.* Now open your eyes and turn your gaze 360 degrees around you. To do this, continue looking as far as you can into the forest, but slowly move your head from front to back in one direction and then the other. In this way get a feel for where you are sitting in relation to the forest that is in your farthest field of vision on all sides. Take your time. When ready, close your eyes and proceed to the next formula.

+ Silently repeat three times *My heartbeat is calm and strong.*

+ Silently repeat three times *My perception is expanding and contracting.* Now open your eyes and focus on a tree that is very close to you. Examine the tree meticulously, the bark, branches, leaves, insect or bird holes, nests, etc. When you have done that, shift your focus out again to the limits of your view and then back to the close tree, and then back and forth a few times. Now explore the areas between your farthest view and immediate surroundings. Gaze at everything around you and at all the varying depths. Try doing this in a causal way—in other words, don't start a methodical search of the area but rather just let your focus rest on whatever draws you. For now keep your focus slowly but continuously shifting from tree to tree at various depths. Forests are perfect for this exercise precisely because they contain naturally spiraling entities—trees—at varying distances and of various proportions, and in moving your focus between them you can saturate your perception in the natural depths of this visual experience. The most important aspect of this exercise is simply to experience the actual reality of depth formed by the relationship of all the living and previously living entities within your field of vision and to actually allow your focus to dance between objects, thus counteracting the perceptual flatness of computer screens, books, and televisions.

Over the course of more than three decades I have spent thousands of hours in tree stands. Some individual trees I have hundreds of hours in. What is so remarkable is that even in those special trees, every time I'm in one I always see new things about the tree and the other trees around it that I didn't see before. When you feel complete in the exercise above, move on to the next portion of the exercise below.

+ Now silently repeat three times *My solar plexus is warm.*
+ Silently repeat three times *The forest is alive with movement.* Now open your eyes and catch the movements of the forest within your visual circle. Everything in the forest is moving—leaves swaying in the breeze, birds flying to and fro, squirrels scampering, twigs dropping, shadows shifting and changing. All these movements and countless others add enormously to the depth of the forest and convert what may ordinarily be viewed as "scenery" into the constantly unfolding process of life. When you feel ready, move on to the next set of formulas.
+ Silently repeat three times *My forehead is pleasantly cool.*
+ Silently repeat three times *I sense everything.* Now open your eyes and realize that from the moment you stepped into the woods, through the time spent getting into the tree and the transition period, right up to the present moment,

you have been submerged in the sounds made both by yourself and those in your environment. Now is the time to focus on the individual sounds within your auditory field. Distinguishing them, and also the distance each source is from you, adds to your perception of the depth formed by the natural environment you are sitting in. Close your eyes for a few minutes (or an hour) and submerge yourself in the auditory reality and depth of the place.

✦ Once you have tuned in to the sounds of the forest, open your eyes and passively place your attention on the smells, colors, textures, shadows, and other qualities of the area and the moment, such as wind, rain, sunshine, or animal movements. By intentionally engaging all of your senses in the various layers of the forest you encounter a depth and quality of experience that far surpasses the flat, mundane, one-dimensional ordinary perception of modern life.

✦ When you are ready, end your session by silently repeating the AT formula *My neck and back are warm.*

✦ While still aware of the area of your neck and back, silently say *I am very quiet.*

✦ Remain relaxed for a minute or two.

✦ Cancel.

By the time you have a few months of experiencing the forest from the depth of perception that the tree stand allows, you will naturally become very sensitive to everything happening within your perceptual field. You probably have started to enjoy the ability to distinguish the sounds of many animals and birds, and your body is becoming accustomed to feeling the different qualities and direction of wind, sun, and rain. When you have reached this point it is time to go completely "under cover" in order to view the forest without being seen or heard. These advanced techniques are divided into three exercises.

Training #28

Advanced Heightened Sensory Awareness and Nature

You begin by setting up your tree stand in a tree that has branches that will camouflage you and making or purchasing a camouflage suit that blends into the forest setting. Hunting outfitters carry a wide range of camouflage patterns for all types of terrain, but if you are going to buy one I recommended getting the reversible-type suit that has two patterns, one for spring and summer foliage and one for fall and winter. It is also important to camouflage your hands and face if you really want to go to the next level. If you are on the ground you can construct a natural blind similar to what duck hunters use, or there are small commercially made camouflage hunting blinds available at sporting goods shops.

This next level begins by staying silent and hidden in your tree stand for long enough periods of time to view the depth of wildlife in the forest. What I mean by "depth of wildlife" is that there are some animals and birds of the forest that are surface dwellers—easily seen, not easily scared, if scared they will return soon, etc., and there are also other classes of animals that won't come anywhere near you if they see you move, smell you, or receive messages that you are there (we will be discussing these "messages" shortly).

The first part of this exercise involves continuing to learn to be absolutely still. This is a skill that requires you to be calm and patient with yourself, to not fidget, to not scratch every itch, to not move your head all around every time you hear or see something. This isn't easy, but the benefits are so rewarding that for many years they took control of my life. A tree stand is absolutely the best way to see wildlife in a forest. The wildlife is not at all expecting you to be silently sitting up in a tree. When you have a great horned owl, wild turkey, hawk, or any type of bird land on a branch just a few feet away from you, or you watch baby deer chasing one another around the base of the tree you are in, you will understand what I mean. I wish I had a dollar for every squirrel that has run up my tree and upon seeing me, gave me the funniest face, as if to say, "What the heck are you doing, you silly human?!" When you have experiences like these you will also understand that seeing these beautiful creatures is just the bonus. The real lesson and prize is the internal calmness and confidence that comes along with these kinds of experiences as you begin to identify with a wider range of species and habitats so far removed from the grimy urban jungle of human beings.

In terms of AT-PM formulas, I suggest doing the same alternating pattern as the previous exercises—one standard, then one PM formula of your choice. For the first part of this advanced technique I just described I would suggest heaviness and warmth formulas, and PM formulas such as *I am invisible, Nothing knows I am here, I'm not here,* or *Nothing can see me.*

The next segment of this advanced exercise is to become aware of the circles within circles of experience and perception that are happening all around you. Every animal and entity in the forest is at once giving off concentric circles of sound, smell, and volumetric information at the same time it is receiving the same sort of information. All of this happens at different levels of intensity and depth. For example, let's start with humans. When you have spent enough time in your tree stand that you are invisible enough to have an owl or hawk land in your tree and stay a while, the flip side of the coin is that you also become painfully aware of how blundering, noisy, and destructive humans are. When the average person steps a few feet into the forest, every living thing runs or flies away. This causes a chain reaction. The animals that are the sentinels of the forest sound the alarm, birds fly away, chipmunks dive into their holes, deer leap into thickets, and squirrels race up trees. Waves of noise and scent are carried off in every direction in widening circles to all the beings in the area. No other animal causes this kind of panicked reaction, but it is important to experience this in order to feel the full effects of how the simple action of a person walking in the woods is carried off in concentric waves of sound out into the forest. Once you are carefully hidden in your tree stand and a person or a domesticated cat or dog comes along, you'll know what I mean.

Once you've experienced the concentric waves given off by modern humans and domesticated animals you'll realize how they don't harmonize with life in a wild setting, but given time, patience, and practice you can begin to feel the different levels of expression and information being given off and received by the various animals and forces that live in the wild. For example, the intensity and type of call made by a blue jay or a crow will send a sound message in a circular pattern out into the forest that other birds and animals recognize and react to. The truth is, animals do talk to one another in myriad ways. If the sounds made by the birds and their patterns of flight indicate the presence of a predator such as a hawk or fox, the other animals that are also wary of hawks or foxes will respond, while other animals who don't feel the threat of the hawk or fox (like deer or bear) are not much affected. When you have experienced this particular sounding of the birds, the reaction of the various other wild animals, and then the actual sighting of the hawk or fox, you will, after a few times of experiencing this, get familiar with the scenario such that you can perceive the concentric circles of information coming to you in a way that you yourself will know when a hawk or fox is coming long before you actually see it.

Perceiving the concentric circles of information that a person is entering the woods is pretty easy; that a hawk is coming is more difficult; that a male deer is on the scent of a female a little harder yet. But the point here is that all of this information is out there, and it takes not some form of extrasensory perception to experience it but rather just treading lightly, being silent, and developing awareness of concentric waves of information, and the doors of perception will open to you in remarkable and healthy ways.

Along with the warmth and heaviness formulas of arms, legs, and back, I like to use the heartbeat formula and especially the solar plexus formula for this technique. I will often use the solar plexus formula many times between other standard formulas.

When you have gleaned the ability to identify concentric circles of information and communication, you are ready to embark on the challenge of engaging the flow. What this involves is entering into a perceptual experience of joining the natural entities and forces around you in both the depth and flow of the living moment. You do this by first throwing away the calendar and forgetting all about what "time" it is in the modern world, and instead focus on what is happening right now in that area of nature in which you find yourself. In a general sense this means feeling the *energy of the season*. Are the trees budding or are the leaves falling? Are the squirrels building nests or collecting nuts? Is it warm or cold, is a storm approaching or maybe one has just passed through? Is the land dry or wet? What birds are around? What are they doing? Which birds are absent? There are countless processes going on in the forest at any given time, and connecting to them can place you into temporal sync with the natural world and away from the abstract rat race where there is never enough "time."

Here is an overview of the training and some PM formulas you might find helpful to use or as models to help create your own:

+ Begin by setting up your tree stand where you are camouflaged by the tree or wear camouflage clothing to blend in.
+ Remain completely still and silent for lengthy periods of time. (I often spend eight to ten hours in my stand with only short breaks every few hours to drink or have a snack.)
+ While still and silent, periodically practice your AT—I like to use the heaviness and warmth techniques here and interject PM formulas between them such as *I am invisible. Nothing knows I am here. I'm not here. Nothing can see me.*
+ Once you have been silent and still enough that animals and birds don't even know you are there, try to perceive the concentric circles of information being sent to you by the forest: animal, bird, and human movement, sounds of leaves rustling, branches falling, or birds calling, smells, etc. The expanding circles of information are all around you—this is your chance to perceive and learn from them.
+ Meld your perception with the energy of the season as described above.
+ This perception and gathering of information is enhanced by AT-PM, so continue using AT practices of your choosing with PM formulas mixed in. At this level of perception my favorite AT practice is the solar plexus. Here are a few PM formulas to use or to help form your own: *I clearly feel the energy of this forest. All my senses are in tune with the flow of this forest. I sense and feel the unfolding of life all around me. I can perceive concentric circles of information coming at me. I am one with the natural rhythm of this forest.*

✦ Please remember to be creative and passively and intuitively craft your own PM
formulas. They are always the finest!

When you successfully meld your perception and the rhythm of
your human organism to the natural flow of the place where you are
sitting, and add that dimension to your full sensory awareness of the
place, you will discover a whole new complete dimension of existence. It
may take months or even years to get to this place, but it is well worth
the trip. The human body and mind have been formed through countless years of being immersed in the primal rhythms and cycles of the
natural world. We are born to relate to the world in this way and to be a
part of the natural flow of life that is continually unfolding around us.
When we engage in a primal awareness of this flow we regain a healthy
sense of temporal reality by leaving behind the one-dimensional feeling
of time imposed by human clocks and calendars. We are able to see and
feel the many dimensions of natural time that are simultaneously being
experienced by the other living beings of the natural world.

12

Primal Connection with the
SENSE OF SMELL

The vast chasm that exists between the way primal peoples view scents and smells and the manner in which we modern people commonly do fascinates me. In terms of understanding primal mind, the sense of smell is extremely illuminating. When I am living with tribal people it becomes apparent right away how much more they rely on scent than I do, and also how much more developed their sense of smell is. Science suggests that during the evolution of the highly intellectual person who relies more on reason than on the senses or instinct, the portions of the brain that govern the senses have given up ground to the intellectual synapses. Of course, unless we have a physical malady or handicap we still have all of our senses, but as is especially the case with our sense of smell, when compared to peoples who use and depend on them daily for survival, we have lost a lot of ground. The good thing is that if we really want to we can reclaim portions of our olfactory acuity. We will be exploring ways to do this, but first let's take a quick look at some intriguing aspects of primal people in relation to scents and odors in order to develop a bigger picture.

CULTURAL VALUES ATTACHED
TO THE OLFACTORY SENSE

In the Andaman Islands between India and Myanmar live the primal Ongee people, considered to be one of the original peoples of India. The Ongee believe that the life force and identifying characteristics of any living being, including humans, resides in their smell. In humans our specific odor emanates from our bones in a similar way that the odor of a plant or tree emanates from its stem or trunk. Personal identity is sensed by catching a whiff of yourself and distinguishing your smell apart from everything else. When Ongee refers to themselves, they touch their noses, which signifies both the olfactory organ and their unique odor.[1]

To the primal Bororo people of Brazil,* the unique smell of a person is a combination of odors from body fluids (associated with the life force) and a person's breath (associated with their soul). By Western standards the Serer Ndut of Senegal have a bizarre belief concerning a person's odor, of which, they say, we all have two. The first is the physical, associated with the body and the breath. The second is the "scent soul" that survives after a person dies, which is reincarnated in a descendant. With this transmigration of scent, the Ndut can tell which dead ancestor is being reincarnated in a child by the similarity of the child's scent with the deceased.

The commingling of odors is taboo in some primal cultures. In the Amazon of the primal Desana people, whom I have had the privilege of visiting extensively on two occasions,† all members of a specific tribe are

---

*One of the anthropologists I respect the most, Claude Lévi-Strauss (1908–2009), lived for some time among the Bororo during his first visits to Brazil. Lévi-Strauss was one of the first anthropologists to argue that the so-called savage (i.e., primal) mind has the same structures as the "civilized" mind, and that human characteristics are the same everywhere.
†In living with indigenous people in Mexico who speak Spanish as a second language I learned to speak it as a second language too. This is extremely helpful when visiting many primal peoples in Central and South America, even though there are differences in dialects. Within many tribes, including the Desana, there are usually men who travel outside the community to trade, and most of these men speak Spanish along with their native tongue.

believed to smell the same. According to the Desana, marriage can only occur between two people with different odors. That means you must marry someone from a different tribe. Other tribes like the Batek in the rainforest of Malaysia don't allow the odors of close relatives to mix, such as in sexual intercourse but also by actually sitting too close to a person with a similar odor for too long.[2] "Watch your back" is a most common theme for the Temiar people, also in Malaysia. One of their beliefs is that your "soul odor" resides in your lower back. If you walk or pass by a person too close, your soul odor can mingle with the other person's and cause illness. Thus when walking or coming up behind a person it is not only customary but imperative to loudly say "ODOR! ODOR!" so that the person's soul odor is prepared to be intruded upon.

It's clear that the taboos of the Desana and Batek serve to discourage inbreeding and encourage diversity by their marrying into other tribes. This also enlarges social ties. If you are Temiar, chances are you won't be taken by surprise by someone coming up behind you! That these cultures associate such important situations as incest, marriage, and soul odor with the sense of smell clearly indicates the high level of value they place on the human olfactory system.

In many cultures food taboos related to odors are prevalent as well. For example, a strict vegetarian people such as the Hindu or Jain of India will be repulsed by the smell of cooking meat, especially beef, as cows are considered sacred, while meat eaters and blood drinkers such as the Maasai of Africa are equally repulsed at the thought of eating greens, as their cattle primarily eat grass. The odors of foods are a primary consideration of what is edible and what is not. Among some primal groups there are even taboos within the simple eating of meat that relate to odor. While living with the Desana in Colombia I found a highly classified system of food preparation in regard to how meat smells. I never found out exactly why, but the Desana relate the smell of burning fat to sexuality. They have strict codes around their sexual customs, and therefore meat is rarely roasted and never fried, thus avoiding the sexually infused odor. Many foods of the Desana are smoked to remove or alter the smell, and then boiled. Through the translations into Spanish I received it appeared to me that the Desana are also highly concerned with what they call "ripeness," which may or may not refer to how ripe a food actually is but also signifies odor. For example, the Desana love to eat small animals and rodents such as agouti (they look like a guinea pig), paca (much bigger than agouti, around two feet long, but look similar), and armadillo. The odor of these animals is said to be "ripe" and therefore safe to eat. Odors of some larger animals such as peccary (called javelina in the United States), tapir, and monkey are considered "overripe" and thus far less desirable. For the Batek, the odor of the animal decides what can be cooked with it. Many meats must have their own fire and are not to be cooked together. Anthropologist Kirk Endicott described a humorous scene with the Batek, in which a woman was "cooking two minnows, three tiny crabs, and two small shrimps over three separate fires!"[3]

Some primal cultures also use odors to stimulate dreams and visions. In Papua, New Guinea, the Umeda men typically sleep with ginger under their heads or their sides. The magic scent of the ginger triggers prophetic visions, many times related to hunting. For an Ongee, whose life-force odor resides in his bones, his spirit while sleeping will leave his body and go to the places he has gone to that day to collect his smell that he left behind and reinsert his odor back into his bones. Without replacing the life-force odor the man would become depleted and eventually die. While participating in an ayahuasca ceremony with the Desana the head shaman reminded me of the four main points of the ceremony: "To make me see and follow my sight. To make me hear and follow the sounds. To make me smell and follow the scents. To make me dream, and follow the ancestors."

One of the most ritual-filled and superstitious activities of primal people involves hunting. Aside from complex rituals and ceremonies designed to honor and "call" the spirits of animals they will hunt, in many cultures odor is also significant to a successful hunt. Some cultures use the sweat lodge, or temazcal, to sweat out human odors, followed by a cold bath or shower. Other cultures commonly use natural masking agents like mud, clay, and aromatic herbs. Another form of masking is the use of urine, which is also employed by modern people for hunting deer and bear. I have done this myself and can personally state that it is not pleasant! The idea is to use the urine of an animal that your prey is not afraid of and doesn't consider a threat. For deer I have used fox urine, mostly on my boots, so the deer don't smell my feet as I walk to my tree stand or blind. During the rut (mating season), urine from a female deer in estrous is often used to lure male deer to within shooting range.

My Desana friends surprised me with two odor rituals that I had to complete before I was allowed to hunt with them. A couple of days before the hunt I was told to eat only specific meats. When hunting strong-smelling animals such as peccaries* and tapir, they only eat smoked meat and smoked peppers so the body will emanate the musky odors that these animals like. They prefer to hunt less smelly animals, for which in preparation for a hunt they only eat boiled foods. Some of the most hardcore traditional hunters will sometimes ingest emetic plants or snort powders to intentionally vomit before the hunt. This is said to rid the body of any remaining human odors. The Desana hunters also made me rub aromatic herbs and certain jungle plants on my body and on my weapons just before the hunt.

EXERCISING OUR OLFACTORY SENSE

There are hundreds more examples of the ways in which primal people relate to smell and the immense significance odor plays in every primal culture. But what does that imply for us? The simplest answer resides in the fact that as modern humans we have largely replaced the sense-related parts of our brain with language and intellectual stimuli, and

---

*Called *javelina* in the American Southwest, they were all around and underneath my house at night in Arizona, and boy, they smell terrible; their stench used to drive my German shepherd crazy.

one of the biggest losers has been our sense of smell. By reintroducing smell into our brain we turn on those primal sites, which I believe can improve our quality of life.

Scientific experiments have shown that with practice the regions of our brain associated with olfaction can be redeveloped and further developed, and that it's even possible to reverse the age-related gray-matter reduction that affects the olfactory regions as we get older. Most of these studies were conducted for the training of perfumers,[4] since in Western culture this is the best (and maybe only) way to make money on people who want to smell good. Amazingly, new research conducted by scientists at Rockefeller University revealed that the human nose is much more sensitive than was previously believed and can distinguish close to a trillion different scents.[5] So how do we awaken our noses (actually, as stated earlier, it's more of a brain thing) and realize our primal abilities?

Well, the only way is to take care of your nose and use it more often. The only thing that separates professional perfumers and people in primal cultures from us ordinary people is the number of hours they dedicate to smelling. It's also no coincidence that many perfumers come from families involved in the fragrance trade, and they are taught to use their nose at an early age. It's the same with primal cultures—they spend their whole lives involved with scents instead of books, computers, and television.

Another way to activate your olfaction is to simply begin to smell aromatic things around you—herbs, tea, coffee, chocolate, olive oil, mangoes piled up at the grocery store, whatever. You can use spices from your cupboard such as cinnamon, cloves, coriander, or vanilla, or you can buy high-quality spices. They are easy to find, are not very expensive, and can be used in your kitchen as well as in your smelling exercises. It sounds simple, but such conscious attempts to smell more and more often translate into plenty of work for your nose and your brain. You can also close your eyes and identify scents. When trying to identify a smell, take short, shallow sniffs rather than one long one. You will notice cats and dogs do this when they are initially smelling something. It increases your ability to pick up a scent. When shopping for food, note that the best-smelling items are, for the most part, what your body craves. When purchasing food items, start selecting those things that smell the best to you. Selecting a rye bread, for instance, and deciding on a cheese to go with it, can best be done by sniffing the aroma of the bread and the cheese and determining which combination has the optimal scent. Of course, what smells the best will be a reflection of what your body needs the most.

INCORPORATING SCENT INTO YOUR LIFE

Aside from intentionally going around smelling things—something that I love to do, is completely safe, and has significant positive effects on your brain even after just a few weeks—we can take this to a whole new level by incorporating the powerfully unique aromas of infused oils and essential oils into our training. Infused oils can be easily made at home or bought cheaply because they don't require the same extractive processes, and they don't require a hard-to-extract oil to make up the bulk of the product as essential oils do. Basically, essential oil is the smell essence that is contained within a plant and has been mechanically extracted for use. Distillation is the common extraction method.

Water: This method is most often employed with flowers such as rose and orange blossoms. In this process the botanical material is completely immersed in water and the mixture is brought to a boil. This method protects the oil extracted to a certain degree since the surrounding water acts as a barrier to prevent it from overheating. When the condensed material cools down, the water and essential oil is separated and the oil decanted to be used as essential oil.

Water and steam: This method can be employed with herb and leaf material. During this process, the water remains below the plant material, which has been placed on a grate while the steam is introduced from outside the main still (indirect steam).

Steam distillation: This method is the most commonly used method for extracting oil from a plant. During this process, steam is injected into the still, usually at slightly higher pressures and temperatures than the above two methods.

In a nutshell, making infused oil is a lot like making tea in your kitchen except instead of steeping an herb in hot water you steep it in (unheated) olive, almond, or grapeseed oil and seal the container, preferably glass, definitely not plastic, allowing it to steep typically for a few weeks.

Unless you want to buy or build a still and do a heck of a lot of work (there are instructions online for DIY stills), you will need to purchase infused oils, which is something I do all the time. There are many ways to use both commercial and homemade oils. My favorite way is to put the scent of a chosen plant or herb into the air around me so I can smell it, which is the main point of this chapter. There are two ways you can do this:

The "old-school" way (the way I do it) is simple—using a candle diffuser. You can buy simple diffusers for under ten dollars, or like anything else there are superfancy and really ornate ones where the sky's the limit on price. Normally these are made from soapstone, terra-cotta, or ceramic; a tea candle is placed inside a lower compartment and above the candle a small dish rests (either as part of the diffuser or a separate dish). You put oil either with or without water in this dish. The heat from the burning candle causes the oil in the dish to vaporize, sending scent throughout the room.

Another way to diffuse scent is with a cold-air diffuser or nebulizer. These operate on the principle of atomization, whereby the oil is forced through a pinhole by a stream of air at high pressure. The result is a microfine vapor that contains all the constituents of the oil in the same balance as the liquid form that remains suspended in the air for some time.

Aside from the benefits of giving our nose and brain a workout with myriad smells, infused and essential oils have many well-known health benefits, which are the basis of aromatherapy (or essential-oil therapy). The National Association for Holistic Aromatherapy describes aromatherapy as "the art and science of utilizing naturally extracted aromatic essences from plants to balance, harmonize and promote the health of body, mind and spirit. It seeks to unify physiological, psychological and spiritual processes to enhance an individual's innate healing process."[6]

Aromatherapy provides a number of proven health benefits (for more on specific oils and their benefits see the list on pages 168 to 175):

Stress relief: Perhaps the most widespread and popular use of essential oil is for stress relief. The aromatic compounds from many different essential oils are known as relaxants and can help to soothe your mind and eliminate anxiety.

Antidepressant: Second to stress relief, essential oils are very commonly used to eliminate feelings of depression, and due to the very complicated side effects of pharmaceutical antidepressants this is a very important application.

Boost energy level: Many essential oils are known to increase circulation, raise energy levels, and generally stimulate the body and mind, without the dangerous side effects of other stimulating substances.

Healing and recovery: As stimulants, many essential oils can help increase the rate of healing throughout the body. This can be due to their ability to increase oxygen and blood flow to wounds as well to their ability to facilitate more internal healing processes like those following surgery or illness. The antimicrobial properties of certain essential oils also help keep the body protected during these delicate healing stages.

Headache: Essential oils can be a wonderful solution that can not only eliminate your current headache but possibly reduce the stress, anxiety, or medical origin of headaches to prevent them in the future.

Sleep aid: Essential oils can help you get to sleep and also help provide you with a more balanced sleep schedule.

Enhanced immune-system function: Essential oils can give a serious boost to your immune system if used properly. The antimicrobial effects, as well as the antifungal and antibacterial effects, can protect you from any number of illnesses and infections that could damage your system. This area of aromatherapy is very popular and widely studied.

Pain relief: Pain relief is one of the most useful applications of essential oils.

How to Make Infused Oils

I first began using infused oils many years before using essential oils, while taking classes on wild medicinal plants. There are several plant-based oils that you can use in making infused oils; these are referred to as carrier oils: sweet almond oil, evening primrose oil, jojoba oil, avocado oil, apricot kernel oil, borage seed oil, olive oil, various nut oils (walnut, pecan, hazelnut), grapeseed oil, and various seed oils (hemp, sesame, sunflower). Aromatic plants such as lavender, rosemary, thyme, and sage make great infused oils, as do peppermint, melissa, chamomile, rose, yarrow, juniper, and pine. Also, plants that have a high level of other fat-soluble components, including fat-soluble vitamins, antioxidants, resins, and saponins, can be extracted by macerating the plant material in oil. Calendula is a good example. When you pick calendula flowers you can feel how resinous and sticky they are, a good sign they will work well in oil. Other suitable plants include comfrey, Saint-John's-wort, viola, plantain, and mullein.

There are several methods for making infused oils:

The Sun Method

Dried or fresh plant material can be used in this method. When using fresh herbs, try to pick them on a dry day, after the morning dew has evaporated. Make sure you pick clean plant material from an area you can be sure has not been sprayed with chemicals or fertilizers. This is particularly important as you are not going to wash the plant material; you want it to be as dry as possible to prevent spoilage, though of course you want to brush off any dirt with a soft-bristled brush.

If using leaves such as comfrey or plantain, it's good to let them wilt overnight to reduce some of the water content, but flowers are best used fresh. Chop fresh leafy herbs finely and lightly, and fill a completely dry jar with the material. I usually use mason jars; they seal well, and depending on how many you get at a time they usually cost just a little over a dollar a jar. It's important to chop the herb first, as it exposes more of the plant to the carrier oil, making for a better infusion. Flowers can be put in whole, while dried herbs will most likely come already cut.

If using fresh herbs you can pour the carrier oil of your choice straight on the plant material, but if using dried material it's nice to warm the oil first to get things going. Fill the jar almost to the brim with oil as any air gaps will promote oxidation and spoilage. Stir the contents with a wooden chopstick or glass stirring rod until all the bubbles have dispersed, and cap with a lid or a piece of kitchen roll held in place with a rubber band. This works well for fresh plant material as it allows moisture to escape.

Leave the bottled mixture on a bright sunny windowsill or in a nice warm spot such as beside the boiler or in an airing cupboard. I prefer infusing oils in the sun, but depending on the time of year the most important thing is to leave the bottle somewhere that is consistently warm; windowsills can get cold at night, which encourages condensation. Stir every day for the first two weeks, then leave the mixture alone to infuse for another two to four weeks, making four to six weeks total preparation time. Some oils are nice to double infuse: leave for three weeks, strain, then fill the jar with fresh flowers, and pour the partially infused oil back on top and repeat the process.

Don't forget to label your jars so you remember when to strain them. Strain through a sieve covered in cheesecloth or a jelly bag. If you used fresh material it is wise to let it stand for a week and check if any water has settled in the bottom of the jar. If so, pour off the oil and discard the water. Bottle the resulting oil, and label and date.

The Heat-Infusion Method

This method is quicker if you need to prepare your oil for more immediate use. For this method a double boiler is recommended, or you can improvise one with a pot and a saucepan, or use a bain-marie, a kind of double boiler that caterers use to keep food warm. A double boiler is basically two pots or pans: a large one that looks a lot like a regular saucepan, and a smaller, shallower pan that nestles inside. Chefs and cooks frequently use double boilers for cooking delicate ingredients that have a tendency to seize or separate over direct heat, as when tempering chocolate, whisking up an egg-based sabayon, or keeping gravy warm.

Fill the bottom pot of the double boiler with an inch or two of water and set the shallow pan on top. Over heat, the water in the bottom pan will begin to simmer and transfer a gentle, steady heat to whatever you're cooking in the pan above. Check the bottom pan every now and then to make sure the water hasn't boiled off and add more water if needed.

Use about 50 to 75 grams of dried herb, or 75 to 100 grams of fresh herb per 300 ml of base oil (300 ml = 20 tablespoons, or 1.25 cups). This is an approximate amount, as some herbs are bigger and fluffier than others. Basically, you want the oil to just cover the dried herb. Place the oil and herbs in a double boiler with a tight-fitting lid over a pan of gently boiling water. Allow to infuse at a continuous heat for two hours, making sure the water does not boil away. Stir every half hour or so, and check the progress of your oil.

Strain and bottle, or repeat the process if you desire a stronger, double-infused oil. Always remember to label and date your products.

You can also heat-infuse your oils using the same ratios described above in covered oven-safe cookware in an oven on the lowest possible temperature.

SOME COMMON ESSENTIAL OILS
AND THEIR USE

My introduction to essential oils came while living in the mountains of Northern California. I was introduced to a friend of a friend who was an herbal healer and aromatherapist who had a small shop in the town where we lived. Her shop was amazing in that she had a vast inventory of organic herbs, oils, teas, candles, tinctures, and salves. Over the course of a couple of years she taught me about the use of essential oils, and I've been hooked ever since. Below is a list of some essential oils with their aromas and description of use. Most of these are easily found in stores that carry essential oils.

Allspice berry: The oil has a warm, spicy-sweet aroma. It is used in spicy or masculine scents. *Benefits:* warming, cheering, comforting, nurturing

Amyris: Also known as West Indian sandalwood, although unrelated to the true Indian sandalwood, this oil has a woody, slightly sweet, balsamic aroma suggestive of sandalwood. *Benefits:* calming (especially for your mind) and stimulates muscle relaxation

Basil: There are many types of basil: linalool basil, exotic basil, and sweet basil. The odor of the linalool type is very green and floral and is most often used in expensive perfumes. The exotic type of basil is stronger, with a hint of camphor. Sweet basil helps reduce indigestion, constipation, and stomach cramps. *Benefits:* clarifying, uplifting, energizing, refreshing

Bay: Bay oil is distilled from the leaves and small twigs of the bay rum tree. It has a powerful, spicy-sweet aroma with a distinctive clove note. It is used to produce bay rum fragrance and as a component of fresh, spicy scents. *Benefits:* clarifying, warming

Bergamot: Bergamot oil is cold-pressed from the peel of the nearly ripe bergamot orange fruit. The aroma of bergamot oil is fresh, lively, fruity, and sweet. It is an excellent deodorizer. *Benefits:* uplifting, inspiring, confidence building

Cardamom seed: The oil has a spicy, camphorlike aroma with floral undertones. *Benefits:* warming, comforting

Carrot seed: This oil is distilled from the seed of the common carrot. Its aroma is dry-woody and somewhat sweet and earthy. *Benefits:* replenishing, nourishing, restoring

Cassia bark: *Cinnamomum cassia,* or Chinese cinnamon, is the spice sold as cinnamon in the United States. Ceylon cinnamon (*Cinnamomum zeylanicum*) is considered the true cinnamon in most of the rest of the world. The oils of both contain cinnamic aldehyde as the major component, with cassia having the larger amount. Caution: Cassia oil is very irritating to the skin and should be handled with care. *Benefits:* comforting, energizing, warming

Cedar, Atlas: The Atlas cedar grows in the Atlas Mountains of Morocco and Algeria. The aroma of Atlas cedar is woody, oily, and slightly animal-like. *Benefits:* stabilizing, centering, strengthening

Cedarwood (red): Red cedarwood essential oil actually comes from a type of juniper known as *Juniperus virginiana,* whose common name is Eastern red cedar. The balsamic-woody aroma of cedarwood oil evokes a feeling of inner strength and centeredness. *Benefits:* empowering, strengthening, confidence building

Chamomile (German): Also known as *blue chamomile,* the oil is deep blue, turning green, then brown with age and exposure to light. The odor is sweet, tobaccolike, and fruity-applelike. *Benefits:* calming, relaxing, soothing

Chamomile (wild): Wild chamomile has a fresh, herbal note and a rich, balsamic, sweet undertone that is very long-lasting. *Benefits:* soothing, nurturing

Cinnamon bark: Also known as Ceylon cinnamon, this is the true cinnamon of world commerce. Its aroma is similar to cassia, or Chinese cinnamon. It is a skin irritant and should be handled with care. *Benefits:* comforting, warming

Citronella: The odor of Ceylon citronella is fresh, grassy, and warm-woody. *Benefits:* purifying, vitalizing

Clary sage: This oil has a spicy, haylike, bittersweet aroma. *Benefits:* centering, euphoric, visualizing

Clove bud: This oil has a powerful, spicy-fruity, warm, sweet aroma. Clove oil is highly irritating to the skin and should be handled with caution. *Benefits:* warming, comforting

Coriander seed: This oil has a delightful fragrance—spicy, aromatic, pleasantly sweet, not unlike bergamot orange. *Benefits:* nurturing, supportive

Cypress: The oil has a refreshing, spicy, juniper and pine-needle-like aroma. *Benefits:* purifying, balancing

Eucalyptus: Of the 300 species of eucalyptus trees in the world, *Eucalyptus globulus* is the best known. Eucalyptus has long been used in topical preparations such as liniments and salves. Cineole is the major constituent. *Benefits:* purifying, invigorating

Fennel (sweet): This oil has a very sweet, earthy, aniselike aroma due to its primary constituent, anethole. *Benefits:* nurturing, supportive, restorative

Frankincense: Various species of frankincense trees grow wild throughout western India, northeastern Africa, and southern Saudi Arabia. The oil is distilled from the gum resin that oozes from incisions made in the bark of the trees. It is spicy, balsamic, green and lemonlike, and peppery. *Benefits:* calming, visualizing, meditative

Geranium (Bourbon): This oil has a powerful, leafy-rose aroma with fruity, mint undertones. Bourbon oil, from the island of Reunion, is considered the finest grade and has the best staying power. *Benefits:* soothing, mood lifting, balancing

Ginger: Ginger oil has a warm, spicy-woody odor. It blends well with spice and citrus oils. *Benefits:* warming, strengthening, anchoring

Grapefruit: Typically cold-pressed from the peel of the common grapefruit, the oil has a fresh, sweet, bitter, citrus aroma. *Benefits:* refreshing, cheering

Hyssop: Historically, hyssop herb was regarded as a sacred plant and was used as a strewing herb and incense to purify holy places. The scent of the oil is reminiscent of the herb—spicy, sweet, woody, and strong. *Benefits:* refreshing, purifying

Jasmine: Great expense goes into producing pure jasmine oil. The flowers must be hand picked before dawn when the essence is at its peak, and large quantities are needed to produce small amounts of oil. *Benefits:* calming, relaxing, sensual, romantic

Juniper berry: This oil is distilled from the dried ripe berry of the juniper tree. It has a fresh, warm, balsamic, woody, pine-needle aroma. *Benefits:* supportive, restoring

Lavandin: This is a hybrid plant, the result of a natural cross-pollination of true lavender and spike lavender. The oil has a woody, spicy-green, camphor aroma. *Benefits:* balancing, clarifying, purifying

Lavender: This oil has a sweet, balsamic, floral aroma. *Benefits:* balancing, soothing, normalizing, calming, relaxing, healing

Lavender spike: The oil from the flowering plant has a fresh, eucalyptus-like aroma, somewhat like a combination of eucalyptus and lavender. *Benefits:* purifying

Lemon: The scent of lemon oil is evocative of the fresh ripe peel. *Benefits:* uplifting, refreshing, cheering

Lemongrass: The oil is distilled from a tropical grass native to Asia. It has a powerful, lemony, grassy aroma. *Benefits:* vitalizing, cleansing

Lime: Two types of lime oil are commonly sold, distilled and cold-pressed. Distilled oil is pale yellow or clear in color, with a perfumey-fruity, limeade aroma. Pressed oil is yellowish to green in color, with a rich, fresh, lime-peel aroma. *Benefits:* refreshing, cheering

Marjoram (sweet): Sweet marjoram is distilled from the leaves and flowering tops of the same plant that produces the culinary herb. The aroma of the oil is warm and spicy, with a hint of nutmeg. *Benefits:* warming, balancing

Marjoram (wild): Wild marjoram oil is not a variety of marjoram but is actually distilled from a species of wild thyme that grows in Spain. The oil has a strong, sweet-spicy, eucalyptus fragrance. *Benefits:* purifying, clarifying

Myrrh: This oil has a balsamic, warm, and spicy aroma. *Benefits:* centering, visualizing, meditative

Myrtle: This is an evergreen shrub that grows wild throughout the Mediterranean. The oil has a distinct, spicy, camphorlike aroma. *Benefits:* clarifying, cleansing

Neroli: This oil is distilled from the flowers of the bitter orange tree. It has a very strong, refreshing, spicy, floral aroma. *Benefits:* calming, soothing, sensual

Nutmeg: Nutmeg essential oil is distilled from whole, dried nutmegs that have been cut into small particles and pressed to remove the fixed oil, known as nutmeg butter. The oil has the characteristic aromatic, volatile, oily-spicy fragrance of whole nutmegs. *Benefits:* rejuvenating, uplifting, energizing

Orange (Mandarin): The floral, neroli-like undertones of mandarin orange are evocative and sensual. *Benefits:* uplifting, cheering, sensual

Orange (sweet): More sweet orange oil is produced than any other citrus oil. Two kinds of sweet orange oil are available, distilled or expressed. Distilled oil is a by-product of juice making and has an inferior aroma. Pressed oil has a lively, fruity, sweet aroma. *Benefits:* cheering, refreshing, uplifting

Oregano: Wild oregano oil has a strong, herbaceous, green-camphoraceous, medicinal top note. The middle note is spicy and medicinal. The dry-out is sweet-phenolic woody and bittersweet. *Benefits:* invigorating, purifying and uplifting

Palmarosa: This oil is distilled from a grass closely related to citronella and lemongrass. The oil has a floral-rose grassy scent. *Benefits:* refreshing

Patchouli: It borders on the exotic and even the name *patchouli* evokes images of heady aromas; dark, rich colors; candlelight; incense; and intrigue. The aroma is very intense; it can be described as earthy, rich, sweet, balsamic, woody, and spicy. *Benefits:* romantic, soothing, sensual

Peppermint: Peppermint oil has a powerful, sweet, menthol aroma that, when inhaled undiluted, can make the eyes water and the sinuses tingle. *Benefits:* vitalizing, refreshing, cooling

Peru balsam: This oil is collected from wild trees along the Balsam Coast of El Salvador. It has a very sweet, balsamic, rich, vanilla-like aroma. *Benefits:* anchoring, strengthening

Pine: Pine oil is distilled from the twigs and needles of the Scotch pine that grows throughout much of Europe and Asia. It has a fresh, resinous, pine-needle aroma. *Benefits:* refreshing, invigorating

Rose: This is one of the oldest and best known of all the essential oils and is associated with love. It is warm, intense, and immensely rich and rosy. *Benefits:* romantic, supportive, gently uplifting

Rosemary: Rosemary is known as the herb of remembrance. The plant produces an almost colorless essential oil with a strong, fresh, camphor aroma. *Benefits:* clarifying, invigorating

Rosewood: This is a tropical tree growing wild in the Amazon basin. It has a sweet-woody, floral-nutmeg aroma. *Benefits:* gently strengthening, calming

Sandalwood: Sandalwood oil has a sweet-woody, warm, balsamic aroma that improves with age. *Benefits:* relaxing, centering, sensual

Spearmint: Spearmint is used to energize the mind and body. *Benefits:* refreshing, cooling, vitalizing

Spruce: Several species of evergreen conifer trees are used to produce this pleasant, balsamic, sweet, evergreen-scented essential oil. *Benefits:* clarifying, vitalizing

Tangerine: Tangerine oil is pressed from the peel of ripe fruit. It is an orange-colored oil with the vibrant fragrance of fresh tangerines. *Benefits:* cheering, uplifting

Tea tree: Tea tree oil, from the leaves of *Melaleuca alternifolia* (it is also commonly known as *melaleuca*), has a long history of use by the indigenous peoples of Australia before it was discovered by the crew of the famous English explorer James Cook, who originated the English common name of the plant. The aroma of the oil is warm, spicy, medicinal, and volatile. *Benefits:* cleansing, purifying, uplifting

Thyme (red): This is the natural essential oil produced from the wild thyme plant. It has an intense, sweet, herbal, spicy-medicinal aroma. *Benefits:* cleansing, purifying, energizing

Vanilla: The aroma is lingering, sweet, and balsamic. *Benefits:* calming, comforting, balancing

Vetiver: This oil is rich, woody, earthy, and sweet. It improves with age. *Benefits:* supportive, grounding

Ylang-ylang: This oil is distilled from the early morning, fresh-picked flowers of the *Cananga odorata* tree. The distillation process is interrupted at various points, and the oil accumulated is removed. The first oil to be drawn off is the highest quality; it is graded "extra" and is an important source of perfume. It has an intense floral, sweet, jasmine-like, almost narcotic aroma. *Benefits:* sensual, euphoric

Training #29
Waking Up Our Primal Sense of Smell

The scents of essential and infused oils can be thought of as the archetypal spirit of plants captured in a jar. These aromas stimulate the brain, and the unique shape of a scented oil molecule is like a key that opens a lock in the olfactory nerve receptors in our nostrils. The impression of the aroma is sent directly and immediately to the limbic system,* where memories are stored and pleasure and emotions are perceived. When stimulated, the limbic system releases chemicals that affect the central nervous system. Serotonin counteracts anxiety, while endorphins reduce pain and affect sexual response.

A highly recommended way to begin using essential oils is to purchase a starter kit (six to twelve bottles). Depending on how many oils are in the set, they usually include some or all of these: eucalyptus, grapefruit, lavender, lemon, lemongrass, lime, patchouli, peppermint, pine, rosemary, spearmint, sweet orange, tangerine, and tea tree. As stated earlier, it is important to make sure the oils are pure and preferably single source, as many companies dilute or contaminate their oils. The company I use is Young Living (www.younglivingabundance.com). Their oils are the finest quality I have found.

Here is the suggested training format and suggestions:

Once you have made (or purchased) infused oils or have purchased

---

*The limbic system supports a variety of functions, including adrenaline flow, emotion, behavior, motivation, long-term memory, and olfaction. Emotional life is largely housed in the limbic system, and it also has a great deal to do with the formation of memories.

essentials oils, they are easy to effectively use with a candle diffuser or some type of atomizer. One way to use the scent of the plant oil is to simply infuse the air with it and go about your business. Having the special scent of a plant wafting through my office as I work, vacuum, or read a book can transform a relatively mundane activity into a ritual.

The same applies for AT. I sometimes simply light my diffuser with some oil to set the mood during my sessions without specifically concentrating on the aroma. However, for this training I suggest that you do concentrate on the specific qualities of the plant scents and intentionally stimulate and activate your primal brain.

You can use AT very effectively to stimulate the limbic system of the brain when you combine AT with the scent of herbs and plants. To begin, I suggest a method we have practiced before, and that is to use standard AT formulas interspersed or alternating with PM formulas; in this case the PM formulas will relate to the scent you are smelling.

Here is a sample AT aroma session:

+ Review the descriptions of oil aromas if you don't already have one in mind and choose an herb, plant, or flower oil essence to work with; start up your delivery device (candle diffuser, atomizer, or whatever).
+ While beginning AT with passive breathing, notice the qualities of the natural aroma.
+ When ready, begin AT: starting with your dominant arm, silently repeat three times *My right* (or *left*) *arm is heavy.*
+ Silently repeat six times *The aroma of the herb* (or *plant*, or *flower*, you can name it or not) *is flowing into me.*
+ Silently repeat three times *My arms and legs are heavy and warm.*
+ Silently repeat six times *The scent is . . . (comforting, grounding, cleansing, relaxing, sensual, uplifting*—whatever the quality of the selected oil is).
+ Silently repeat three times *My heartbeat is calm and strong.*
+ Silently repeat six times *The scent is firing up neurons in my brain.*
+ Silently repeat three times *My solar plexus is warm.*

+ Silently repeat six times *I can feel the* (whatever specific feeling or emotions the aroma provides for you personally, e.g., *clarifying*) *energy of the aroma.*
+ Silently repeat three times *My forehead is pleasantly cool.*
+ Silently repeat six times *The scent messages are flowing through my body.*
+ Stay with the feelings of the aroma and silently repeat three times *My neck and back are warm.*
+ Before canceling, stay with the aroma for as long as you wish.
+ Remember how the herb, plant, or flower scent affected you.
+ Cancel.

Remember, the above is just a sample exercise and a good place to start, but the formulas you come up with on your own are endless. Also, it is very effective to replace the standard formulas with other formulas such as healing formulas, affirmations, or any others that you choose. Throughout the years I have developed relationships with specific aroma essences that I use for specific situations. In the beginning it is enjoyable to experience trying various aromas and discovering which ones work best for you. Here are a couple of final thoughts:

• Some herbs, flowers, or plants I say by name out loud during AT. These are usually ones that I know or have picked myself. But using a plant's name can sometimes be distracting. For example, sniffing lavender for a guy seems kind of effeminate or "girly" for those who think that way. If you didn't know the scent was lavender you might feel differently about it. In my case my female partner loves lavender, and I love it when she has it on her. Distractions can also occur in relation to oil names we aren't familiar with, such as ylang-ylang, vetiver, neroli, or patchouli. In any case it's certainly not necessary to name a plant, an herb, or a flower when working with its aroma. Sometimes, unless you are familiar with it, it's best not to name it.

• Be prepared for memories to pop up when you smell aromas you are already acquainted with. In my case there is simply no way that I won't think of my partner when I smell lavender. So the only time I use it is when I want to think of her. This can actually be very helpful if I'm traveling for long periods of time and I miss her. But unless I intentionally want to think of her I wouldn't use lavender during my AT session. If you have fond memories of a place in nature or of a person who wears a specific natural scent you can use it to think of that place or person, however, if you have had not very good associations with any plant aromas (maybe an ex?), be prepared or stay away. Scents are powerful in developing and also recalling memories because of their potent action on the limbic system.

MAKING HERBAL BODY BUTTER

Maybe it's just because I'm a man, or maybe because I'm a man who grew up in semirural areas (when I was in junior high my school was closed on the first day of deer-hunting season), but for whatever reason I never understood why someone (especially a man) would want to rub a cream on their entire body. I thought I would just feel sticky and greasy and who wants that? But I admit now that I was wrong.

As we saw earlier, primal people have been rubbing herbs and plants and all kinds of smelly and sticky concoctions on themselves for millennia. What I learned from my friend, the master herbalist, is that the trick to not feeling sticky or greasy is to use a high-grade herbal butter and apply it at the right time (more on that later). My herbalist friend gave me a jar of such an herbal butter—I think it was rosemary-infused (one of my favorites)—and I had really great experiences with it. The simple act of rubbing and infusing the smell of the spirit of the plant into my skin opened primal nose-brain pathways that were long dormant. Needless to say, I was very surprised and thrilled. However, when I used it all up and went to buy a jar I almost choked at the price. So I basically begged my friend to teach me how to make herbal butter. Turns out it's not difficult, it's much cheaper than buying it, and it's well worth the time.

These are the simple ingredients I use to make herbal body butter (of course there are many other ways you can try):

- **½ cup shea butter:** Shea butter is sourced from the seed of the shea tree of West Africa (*Vitellaria paradoxa*). It has anti-inflammatory properties, protects against sunburn, and can aid in healing minor cuts and abrasions. It is also incredibly moisturizing. It's edible and has been used for millennia as a traditional African food source, but it's not tasty.
- **¼ cup coconut oil:** Coconut oil is the oil extracted from the meat of matured coconuts. It is antiviral, antimicrobial, antibacterial, and it protects against sunburn, blocking about 20 percent of harmful UV rays. It is also very moisturizing. Edible and tasty.
- **¼ cup jojoba oil:** Jojoba oil is a liquid wax (not really an oil) derived from the seed of the jojoba plant native to southern Arizona and California, and northwestern Mexico. It has antiviral, antibacterial, and anti-inflammatory properties. It seals in the skin's moisture. Edible but noncaloric and nondigestible.
- **Essential or infused oil:** Five to ten drops of essential oil, more if using infused oil. For the herbal body butter I prefer essential oil because you don't need very much. The quantity needed to get a good aroma from infused oil can make the butter a little bit slimier.

As when making infused oil you will need a double boiler. For this herbal butter I recommend a relatively shallow top pan, which will make it easier to whisk the ingredients.

How to Make Herbal Body Butter

✦ Put a couple of inches of water in the bottom pan. Place shea butter, coconut oil, and jojoba oil in the top pan. Turn on the heat.

✦ Over medium heat, whisk the oils together until they are melted and combined. Mixture will go from white to semiclear when ready.

✦ Refrigerate melted oils for an hour or until white and solid.
✦ With an electric stand mixer or a hand mixer, beat the oils until they are fluffy, like whipped cream.
✦ Add essential or infused oils, and beat to incorporate.
✦ Fill your desired container(s) with the whipped herbal body butter, and refrigerate another hour.

It's best to rub in a light layer of the herbal body butter just after a hot shower, while the pores of your skin are still open. It may feel a little greasy immediately after application, but within minutes it will soak into your skin. This body butter will keep about six months at room temperature. It may soften in warm weather because of the coconut oil.

Training #30
Herbal Body Butter

AT sessions with herbal butter are relaxing and informative and can be highly addictive! I suggest using formulas in a similar way with the oils but with one addition: It's very effective to rub the oil in while performing a standard formula related to that body part (arms, legs, solar plexus, etc.). I also sometimes use the energy tunnel locations while rubbing the oil in, but in this case instead of visualizing color, visualize aroma. For example, in the oil aroma sample formula I say to myself *My limbic system is sending the scent messages throughout my body.* While rubbing in your scented butter you could be more specific and say *My limbic system is sending the scent energy to my abdomen* (or any other specific tunnel or associated organ like your heart, neck, thyroid, thymus, third eye, solar plexus, or abdomen—the sky is the limit). And guys, you can do this at home in private and not tell your buddies.

✦ After a nice warm/hot shower or bath have some room temperature or slightly warmer herbal butter ready.
✦ Review the qualities of the plant used to make the butter. For example, if you

used lavender you have made a butter that is balancing, soothing, normalizing, calming, relaxing, and healing.

+ Choose an AT formula you simply feel comfortable with or one more that resonates with qualities of the plant. With lavender I would probably choose formulas relating to the balance of the sixth tunnel or standard formula #7— cooling the forehead. This is also a good time to practice affirmations.

+ With these considerations in mind—gently rub the magical energy of the butter into your skin while performing your chosen AT practice(s) and affirmations. And most of all—enjoy!

13

Primal Connection with the

WORLD OF NATURE

We have a history of millions of years of relating to wilderness, literally and bodily . . . Entering the wilderness and its microcosms gives us an opportunity to reconnect with that instinct and rests our fragile psyches from the exhaustion of trying to stay intact in the civilized world, which is so alien to many of us. . . . Merger with a therapist can heal our abandonment wound, but merger with nature can reconnect us to the ancient roots of the Self as well. . . . The healing that comes to me from being in the wilderness is the opportunity to leave ordinary consciousness and return to my animal, instinctual way of being.[1]

The above quote is from a book written by a mother-daughter team of psychotherapists who inspire urban dwellers toward an awareness of primal mind through participation with nature. On the other hand there are many people, such as famous actor, writer, and director Woody Allen, who feel quite the opposite. Allen once said, "Nature and I are two." Perfectly comfortable in his hometown of New York City, Mr. Allen is noted for taking extraordinary, and comedic, precautions to stay away from nature, saying he never goes into natural lakes because "there are living things in there."[2]

The first quote by the Wheelwrites is a perfect example of what ecopsychologists are now referring to as *biophilia*, which "boldly asserts the existence of a biologically based, inherent human need to affiliate with life and lifelike processes. This proposition suggests that human identity and personal fulfillment somehow depend on our relationship to nature. The human need for nature is linked not just to the material exploitation of the environment but also to the influence of the natural world on our emotional, cognitive, aesthetic, and even spiritual development."[3]

Aversion to nature—what some ecopsychologists term *biophobia*—is increasingly common among people raised with television, computers, iPods, and video games, who live in a world of shopping malls, freeways, and dense urban and suburban settings where nature is only accessible as tasteful decoration. These folks tend to avoid or even scorn things that are not man-made and environments that are artificially maintained. So now the question arises: Is aversion to nature simply one of many equally legitimate ways to relate to nature? For me and all the others actively pursuing more holistic lifestyles in accordance with healthy environments, the answer is a resounding NO! Our natural world supports biophobes, biophiliacs, and everyone in between. The problem with biophobia, however, is what economists call the "free-rider" syndrome. A free-rider is someone who partakes of the benefits of action against a problem but doesn't take part in the action itself. In terms of nature and environmental issues, biophobic free-riders benefit from those fighting for clean air (which they breathe), clean water (which they drink), preservation of biological diversity (which sustains them), and conservation of soil (which feeds them). Biophobia is not a sustainable way of life, and it unfairly distributes the work of keeping the earth (as well as any local place) healthy for everyone.

The great chasm between the notions of biophilia and biophobia didn't just happen overnight; it occurred like a slow tectonic shift in attitudes through the late Middle Ages to the present moment. These are very complex situations we are now dealing with. For example, what about people who are basically averse to nature but donate to environmental organizations like the Sierra Club because they like the *idea* of nature? I'll use myself as an example, because in many ways I am a hypocrite too. I am a tried-and-true biophiliac, but I still own a car. I spend way more time in nature than most people, but currently I don't live off the grid like I used to, so right now I'm sitting in front of my computer, which is powered (at least partially) by a nuclear power plant.

For me, the key issue is balance. We are all free-riders at one level or another. It's not a matter of judging one another, but a good idea would be to educate one another. Right now in human history we are way off balance on the side of technology and consumption. It is my belief that in reconnecting with the complex processes of our human organism through AT, while also reconnecting with our larger body, which is primal mind/nature, we rekindle our sense of wonder, which in turn helps us expand the view of our place in this world. Reconnecting with nature and our body also helps us regain awareness of primal mind in ways that support psychophysiological health and wellness.

With that in mind I have dedicated the next two chapters of this book to specifically combining AT and nature-based trainings to provide primal-mind experiences that arise from nature. One of my favorite aspects of AT is that you can practice anywhere and with anything. AT-PM experiences with nature are amazing opportunities for personal growth, and I hope you "dig" them as much as I do.

Training #31
Forest Bathing and the Nature Bed

Researchers in Japan have finally found something I have long been waiting for: scientific evidence that spending time in a forest is good for your health! Medical doctors and scientists have proven that "forest bathing," i.e., intentionally spending quiet time in a forest, lowers stress levels, has positive effects on our physical, emotional, and mental well-being, and can even help a person fight cancer. *Shinrinyoku,* or forest bathing, was introduced in 1982 in a prescient move by the Forest

Agency of Japan to encourage a healthy lifestyle and decrease stress levels. Forest bathing has now become a recognized relaxation and stress management activity in Japan. As an unexpected bonus, studies conducted in the last few years show that forest bathing also increases a component of the immune system that fights cancer.

Qing Li, a senior assistant professor at Nippon Medical School in Tokyo, is currently the president of the Japanese Society of Forest Medicine, which was established in 2007. Dr. Li has conducted a number of experiments to test the effects of forest bathing on mood, stress levels, and immune function. In one study, the profile-of-mood-states (POMS) test was used to show that forest bathing significantly increased the score of vigor in test subjects and decreased scores for anxiety, depression, and anger—leading to the recommendation that habitual forest bathing may help to decrease the risk of psychosocial stress-related diseases.

Other studies on immune function looked into whether forest bathing increases the activity of natural killer (NK) cells, the component of the immune system that fights cancer. In two studies, a small group of men and a small group of women were assessed before and after a two-night/three-day forest-bathing trip. During the trips the subjects went on three forest walks and stayed in a hotel in the forest. Blood tests were taken before and after the trip, revealing a significant boost in NK activity in the subjects in both groups. The increase was observed as long as thirty days after the trip. Follow-up studies showed a significant increase in NK activity was also achieved after a day trip to a forest, with the increase observed for seven days after the trip. Dr. Li attributes the increase in NK activity partly to breathing in air containing phytoncide (wood essential oils) like α-pinene and limonene, which are antimicrobial volatile organic compounds emitted from trees to protect them from rotting and insects.

Although in Japan 67 percent of the land is still forested and easily accessible, Dr. Li says forest bathing is possible anywhere in the world where there is a patch of decent forest (generally defined as land with a tree canopy cover of more than 10 percent in an area of more than half an acre). He says that while forest bathing it's not important that we do heavy physical exercise; rather, one should "enjoy the forest through the five senses: the murmuring of a stream, bird's singing, green colour, fragrance of the forest, eat some foods from the forest and just touch the trees."[4] For those of us lacking the time or resources to forest bathe, Dr. Li says a two-hour walk in a city park with a good density of trees can significantly boost the score for vigor and decrease symptoms of anxiety and depression.

Of course, those of you who are familiar with my previous books know that I have been saying this for decades. So here I'm going to introduce a simple but powerful training that combines the primal mind of forest bathing, AT, and a practice known as "The Nature Bed." This training can be done alone or with a partner or in a group. One nature bed can be used with a partner or small group, each person contributing to the creation of the bed. With larger groups multiple beds are more suitable.

+ Go to an attractive place in nature that is relatively flat and has an open area large enough for you to lie down in with your arms stretched out from your sides. The whole landscape need not be flat; you could be in a hilly or mountainous region; it's just that where you lie down should be flat simply for comfort.

+ Now delineate a circle just large enough in which to lie down inside with outstretched arms. This can be done in many ways depending on the land. You could use sticks, leaves, rocks, pinecones, or whatever is naturally around you to mark the borders of a circle.

+ Once you have a circle, "clean" the inside by gently removing rocks, sticks, or anything else that could poke you when you lie down. Anything that you remove from inside the circle carefully place on your line of delineation.

+ Next, gather leaves, pine boughs, grass, or whatever is around you and place them inside your circle to make a comfy bed. Do your best to make it aesthetically pleasing as well. Depending on the time of year I have participants in my workshops decorate the bed with flowers, so you can also do this if you like.

We only take the lives of plants or flowers for special reasons or for food. If you take flowers, simply explain to them that it is your desire to connect with them and that their energy will have far wider implications as you walk the earth with their spirit inside you.

+ Weather permitting, remove your shoes as you enter the circle, then lie down on your back with arms to the sides, palms touching the earth.

+ For the next ten minutes or for as long as you like simply lie in your bed and feel the energy of the place in nature where you are. Each place in nature has a unique quality and feeling. Try to tap into the personality of the place where you are. During this period I like to close my eyes to better feel the earth on my back and palms and also open them to see leaves and branches moving, birds flying, clouds moving, etc.

+ When you are ready, proceed into AT. I'm going to give you the following session as an example, but of course you can modify it if you like.

+ Engage in two minutes of passive breathing, silently repeating *I breathe me.*

+ Passively focus on each of the areas below, one at a time:

+ Starting with your dominant arm, silently repeat three times *My right* (or *left*) *arm is heavy.*

+ Here inject your own formula related to the place (e.g., *The forest breathes me*). Silently repeat this six times.

+ Silently repeat three times *My heartbeat is calm and strong.*

+ Here inject your own formula related to the place (e.g., *The breeze* [or *air*] *caresses me*). Silently repeat this six times.

+ Silently repeat three times *My solar plexus is warm.*

+ Here inject your own formula related to the place (e.g., *I am part of the living soil*). Silently repeat this six times.

+ Silently repeat three times *My arms and legs are warm.*

+ While still aware of the warmth in your arms and legs, say to yourself *I am very quiet.*

+ Remain relaxed for a minute or two.

+ Cancel.

+ Repeat this sequence two more times.

+ During your second and third cycle, spontaneously change your free-form formulas (or your standard formulas) based on your feelings, sensations, and emotions, but remember, it's always best to end with one of the standard body-centered formulas for grounding.

When finished, take your circle apart while reflecting on your experience and thank the place for its gifts of sharing. Put the place back the same as it was before you came or at least to the point where no one would know you had been there. While doing this, realize that whatever you just experienced, whether profound or not, undoubtedly touched some level of your primal mind just by the setting and your actions. The level of depth into your primal mind depends on how far you let yourself embrace the exercise.

Training #32
The Multidimensional Primal Relationship—Predator and Prey

The relationship between predator and prey is a never-ending cycle in nature. Disconnection from our food sources, domestication of animals, and living in temperature-controlled environments has effectively removed us from these cycles to an extent that most people in urban environments live their entire lives without ever personally witnessing the natural process of predator and prey. Fish eat other fish, insects eat insects, and even some birds eat other birds. Sure, there are animals that eat mostly or only plants, but even many of these herbivores are prey for other animals.

All beings of the earth are connected through the cycle of predator and prey. That includes humans too, but at this point in time we humans are primarily at the top of the food chain, picking and choosing which plants and animals are most profitable and convenient to exploit for our food. Of course, there are people who eat only plants, but even those people are part of the life cycle as well, for even animals at the top of the food chain—eagles, lions, and humans—are ultimately prey for the Great Huntress. This Great Huntress, whom we know as death, makes all things equal. The one inevitable consequence of all life is death, and sooner or later we each become the prey of she who shows us our mortality and returns our body to the earth to complete the cycle.

This should not feel like a morbid concept. The cycles of life and death and predator and prey are interwoven within the balance of life on Earth. Awareness of that one sure moment that will come in your life can give your life strength and immediacy. The skills of predation and escape make all animals what they are. This includes not only hunting skills but survival skills as well. The smartest, strongest, and most alert beings survive. Animals develop skills and grow strong and knowledgeable while trying to evade the predator and live to see another day. In this respect, however, humans have become weak. Our modern pursuits have advanced us in other areas, but at the cost of our wildness and the abilities and skills of our primal mind pertaining to survival in the world of nature and wilderness.

In this training we will attempt to enter our primal mind and, without actually killing anything, delve into both sides of the predator-prey relationship. In doing so we will discover and explore feelings and skills that are inherent to the cycle of life. This training will require you to cultivate an inner attitude of being both predator and prey, to explore what it feels like to be engaged in the covert search for prey, and also the awareness that just around the bend you might find yourself being prey for a larger or more skillful predator.

The following is a sample AT session geared specifically for this training, which you can customize or modify. If at all possible, for this training it is best to locate yourself in an area of wilderness that is full of animal life—a forest in the nonwinter months is ideal.

✦ This training begins the moment you first enter the woods. Notice what happens when a human enters the woods—everything else scatters. Birds fly away, deer run off, squirrels scamper up trees, the insects stop buzzing. It's kind of sad but true: the only thing we can do if we want to see any wildlife is find a nice spot and be quiet and still for a while. So that's what we're going to do. Walk as far as you feel comfortable while looking for a spot that calls to you, and then sit down and be very still.

+ Since we are totally silent when we do AT this is the perfect time to begin.

+ Engage in two minutes of passive breathing, silently repeating *I breathe me.*

+ Passively focus on each of the areas below, one at a time.

+ Starting with your dominant arm, silently repeat three times *My right* (or *left*) *arm is heavy.*

+ Here inject your own formula related to a predatory animal, silently repeating it six times; for example, *I am the wolf that stalks the forest.*

+ Silently repeat three times *My heartbeat is calm and strong.*

+ Here inject your own formula related to an animal of prey (e.g., *I am a squirrel always attentive*). Silently repeat it six times.

+ Silently repeat three times *My solar plexus is warm.*

+ Here inject your own formula related to a predatory animal (e.g., *I can smell my prey is near*). Silently repeat it six times.

+ Silently repeat three times *My arms and legs are warm.*

+ Here inject your own formula related to an animal of prey (e.g., *Always vigilant, always vigilant*). Silently repeat it six times.

+ Silently repeat six times *My neck and back are warm.*

+ While still aware of the warmth in your neck and back, say to yourself *I am very quiet.*

+ Remain relaxed for a minute or two.

+ Cancel.

+ Repeat this sequence at least two more times. During your second and third sequence spontaneously change your free-form formulas (or your standard formulas) to foster visceral feelings of being both the predator and the prey.

+ After your last cancel, get up and begin walking as slowly and quietly as you can. While walking, transform your perception into that of the predator. You are a pure predator hunting the woods with skill and precision. You notice everything that moves, everything that breathes, and every shape and color and pattern that surrounds you. You move silently, keeping your own sounds to a bare minimum while you listen and process every natural sound around you. Listen attentively for any sounds of the movement of prey or signals in the air that clue you in to the presence of your prey. Feel with all of your senses and intuition what is happening around you as you continue to walk slowly through the forest.

+ The moment you see or hear a living being it becomes your prey. Avoid being seen or heard by your prey as you approach it. Crouch behind trees or bushes and time your movements with the wind or other sounds. Keep the feeling of being the predator inside of you as you stalk your prey. As soon as you see your prey it is yours. There is no need to try to catch it; get as close as you can or simply move on to your next target.

+ Explore deeply the feeling of being a skilled predator while stalking in this way for a minimum of half an hour (an hour or two is even better). Then switch to the sense of being the prey of something infinitely stronger and smarter than you. Feel deeply and at the core of your being that you are suddenly being watched. There is something out there that is highly skilled and deadly silent, and it is after you. Notice every sound around you; see every movement in the environment as a potential threat. Continue walking with this primal feeling. Where is it? Where is your pursuer hiding, from which direction is it coming?

+ Try to maneuver in a way that your hunter can't predict. Be calm but hyperaware. Put your primal mind into overdrive. Use everything available to you to conceal yourself as you steal stealthily along. Walk in the shadows, hide momentarily behind trees or bushes, at times walk while crouching low to the ground, or crawl, watching everything around and above you. It is no good if you stop moving; you must keep moving or you will be caught. Explore this feeling of being the prey for at least half an hour.

+ To end the training, try exploring the feeling of simultaneously being both predator and prey. This is the condition of most animals in the wild—the endless pursuit of food coupled with the threat of becoming the food of another creature at any instant. Explore this dual feeling deeply while walking in the forest, and you will better understand the cycles of life in the natural world.

There are many ways of enhancing the experience of this training. One way would be to imagine yourself as a specific animal. For example, if you are walking as the predator and you spot a squirrel, you might try transforming your perception into that of a large cat or a bird of prey such as a hawk stalking the squirrel. Walking with this feeling of being one of the real-life predators of the animal world can really help you cultivate a more intense experience. Or vice versa, you could feel yourself as a mouse and that an owl or fox is hunting you. The idea is to simply explore as fully as possible the aspects of both sides of the coin, and then both at once. Open up to letting the actual place of nature enhance your experience by supplying the sounds, movements, colors, textures, shadows, smells, and animals that will provide you with a powerful experience of a primal nature.

Training #33

Nature's Breath

This training puts us in touch with the primal connection we have to vegetation and trees, which provide an essential key to being alive—oxygen for our breathing.

+ Find a tree or a green plant. A potted plant will do, but an attractive place in nature is even better.
+ Sit down comfortably with the tree or potted plant, and perform an AT session.
+ Engage in two minutes of passive breathing, silently repeating *I breathe me*.
+ Passively focus on each of the areas below, one at a time.
+ Starting with your dominant arm, silently repeat three times *My right* (or *left*) *arm is heavy*.
+ Silently repeat six times *I breathe this tree* (or *plant*).
+ Concentrate on your heartbeat and silently repeat three times *My heartbeat is calm and strong*.
+ Silently repeat six times *I breathe this tree* (or *plant*).
+ While still aware of your breath, say to yourself *I am very quiet*.
+ Remain relaxed for a minute or two.
+ Cancel.
+ Repeat this sequence two more times. On your last cancel, open your eyes, stand up, and stare intently at the tree or plant and stop breathing (hold your breath). At the moment you stop breathing, say to yourself *I breathe you* over

and over, again noticing how disconnected to the web of life you are in that moment because you are not breathing. Notice how the suffocating feeling is so unnatural and out of tune with your body and mind.

✦ Only when you have to begin breathing again while hugging the tree or touching the plant, acknowledging that it produces the oxygen you need to survive. Notice how awesome and primal it feels to be breathing again.

✦ Repeat one or more times, with or without the AT session.

✦ When back indoors, try this exercise without the AT session, using an unnatural object such as a TV or microwave. I'm serious! Silently say to your fridge or couch *I breathe you*. Actually do it, and see how you feel about both the indoor item and the tree or plant.

Training #34
Temporary Shelter

Reawakening and expanding our senses, along with many techniques relating to nature, can help reintroduce us to our primal mind and counteract in a positive way many of our narrow views and experiences of spending so much of our lives indoors. Spending time in a temporary shelter out in nature can help counteract the effects of ecologically traumatizing technology and lifeless artificial permanent structures. This implies living for a period of time in a debris hut, tent, yurt, teepee, or some other kind of structure that is impermanent or portable and that contains little or no modern technology. Engaging in this type of experience is not merely some form of romanticizing what life used to be like before technology or an attempt to recreate such lifestyles; it is more of a process of discovering what we have lost *and* gained by our technology so that we can claim knowledge of more appropriate uses for what we know and have.

It is easy to list the ways that technology has made our lives more comfortable, but sometimes this perceived comfort masks many of the benefits that have been lost by the old way of doing things, especially when viewed from the perspective of how we relate to the natural world at the most basic, primal level. Take, for example, central heating, which most of us rely on to stay warm. Prior to the advent of heating with fossil fuels and electricity (often supplied by nuclear power plants), people relied on heat from a fire, whether a woodstove, hearth, or campfire. Fire in this case was not just a source of heat but was also the center of a plethora of social, physical, and psychological activities. Firewood needed to be collected, cut, and stacked, typically with each household member contributing to the work. The sparking of the morning fire marked the start of a new day, and in the evening fire was the center of the evening meal, a place where food was cooked as well as a place around which family members gathered for warmth, discussions, storytelling, music, and sharing.

This example is given not to simply arouse romantic feelings of the good old days or to suggest that we all use wood for heat. I use it to shed light on the fact that technology, which in this case is a central heating system, has replaced not just an elemental source of heat but also a whole set of relationships and circumstances that for millennia were central to human life and community. The simple wood fire connected us to the local landscape as well as to one another. Today the home-heating furnace, as well as all the pipelines, oil tankers, and everything else that is part of the fossil-fuel industry has replaced whole worlds of relationships, reducing them to the setting of a thermostat and the monthly paying of a bill.

This same situation applies to many of our technologies. Whereas once we related to the world in a visible, give-and-take manner, now we simply push a button, turn a knob, or look at a flat screen. All this happens, for the most part, with technology operating behind the scenes, without our ever seeing it, let alone knowing how it works. We know how to turn knobs and push buttons, but most of us really have no idea how the specific technology we are using actually works. This is part of the great promise of technology—to alleviate us from the burdens of life. But so many of these so-called burdens aren't burdens at all; they are actually necessary experiences that ground us and connect us to life. When we disconnect from these life-affirming experiences we reduce some of the most important aspects of living to commodities and products.

The primal training I will introduce here is that of living in a temporary or impermanent structure that places you squarely in the natural world with a minimal layer of padding between you and nature. The exercise is quite simple. First, make the arrangements necessary to spend at least a few days (a week or longer is even better) living out of your impermanent structure. The more time you spend in and around your structure, the more you will get from this practice. In other words, try to avoid going into your house or any other permanent buildings as much as possible. Figure out alternatives to meet your basic needs. The level that you do this at will depend entirely on your personal situation, but the idea is to fully embody the exercise and push your limits of creativity, patience, and discipline.

This type of experience forces you into reevaluating everything in your life, starting with the simplest things like: How will I go to the bathroom? How will I stay warm and dry? What will I eat? Facing these realities opens our eyes to all of the circumstances and experiences of the natural world that we insulate ourselves from by almost always being inside, and it also brings to light many of the activities and skills that have been lost through our dependence on technology and machines.

Where and how to do this training: For those of you with experience in camping with a tent (not in a motor home), I suggest you go another step forward (or in this case, backward) and make yourself a natural shelter or debris hut. There are many books and plenty of online resources that detail how to do this. If you haven't camped outdoors before, you will probably (but not necessarily) want to use a tent. Borrowing one from a friend is fine if you yourself don't own one. Purchasing one is another option, but I suggest that if you're going this route do some research and look at different types of tents. Well-made tents can last a long time, so it's best to buy one that will fit your needs after this training. I have had my single-man tent for over thirty years; I've used it countless times, and it's still in great shape. Bigger tents don't seem to last as long (at least for me), mainly because they're higher and wider so they have more surface area for wind and other elements to strike at. Another option is to use a temporary, portable structure such as a tipi or yurt. I have spent significant time living in both of these. I had my own tipi for many years and have friends who have yurts. If you know someone who has either one of these circular structures they are great to spend time in.

Simply sleeping on the ground in a sleeping bag can be a very powerful primal experience. Many years ago when I began sleeping on the ground when I stayed among primal peoples my life changed radically. One year when I was writing instead of traveling, I would spend parts of the day inside (with frequent short walks in the woods with my dog) on the computer,* and then I would spend the night outside in my tent simply because I liked it so much. I slept better on the ground, with the sounds and smells of nature around me, the moon and stars above me.† Even though my tent was only a short walk from my house, that year I slept outside in my tent for over 290 days out of 365, and the experience made me a more well-rounded person.

Choose a place in nature where there's little chance of being disturbed. If you know someone who owns some land out in a rural setting, that would be ideal, or you could simply ask permission from a landowner, something I have done on several occasions with positive results. Just be sure that whatever location you choose it's legal for you to be there, as the worst thing is to have a game warden or forest ranger come walking into your camp. Also, and this may seem self-evident: be sure to choose a time of year that will be comfortable for you to try this training. We're not trying to push ourselves beyond our survival

---

*Because I prefer to write outside, weather permitting, I have a homemade "shelter" for my laptop. Basically, it's a three-sided box with a roof made of plywood that my laptop fits inside of so that I can work without the glare of the sun. I just sit this computer shelter on a table, place the laptop inside, and do my writing.

†I have a few different types of tents, each designed for different types of weather and different numbers of people. My lightweight tent has a mesh roof so I can see the stars. It has a rainfly to put over the mesh in case it rains.

limits here. The goal is to get out of the house and into nature for a longer period of time than just taking a hike, but we also need to be safe. Don't go too far into the wilderness, and make sure to tell someone exactly where you will be (or better yet, show them).

Bring with you what you need, but don't go overboard. Leave your electronic toys at home. Your temporary structure should be about as opposite of your house or apartment as possible. Sleeping bag, pillow, flashlight, food and water, a good book—all these are fine. If you know how to make a campfire safely, bring material for making one.

Only you can decide the exact format of this training. How much time you have, your outdoor skill level, the time of year, where to be, etc.—it's all up to you.

Spending time in a temporary shelter affords you plenty of quiet time for practicing AT, visualization, meditation, and the nature trainings that are included in this chapter. Fresh air and only the sounds of nature around you provide a healthy and novel atmosphere for the trainings in this book. Whether inside my shelter or just outside of it, some of my favorite trainings include the advanced visualization techniques outlined in trainings 13 through 16 (chapter 8). The visualization of people, abstract concepts, self-participation, and self-directed questions seems to flow even better when I'm alone outside in a safe environment. When we are away from our regular routines and our physical possessions we afford ourselves opportunities for learning in new environments. These can provide us with an expanded view of ourselves and our place in the world.

Training #35
Feeling in the Dark

Since I was a youngster I've been fascinated by the art and process of photography. I went to college for photography and after graduating I apprenticed with some well-known photographers before starting my own business. During my apprenticeships I spent *a lot* of time in the darkroom developing negatives and making prints. Aside from the technical skills I was learning, a powerful by-product of that time was the development of my primal ability to work in darkness. Without being able to see, all of my other sense faculties were engaged and heightened.* Thus in my daily life it became quite natural to do things in the dark that most people don't or won't do. Some people might say, "Big deal, why don't you just turn on a light?" Well, that's a good point, but what I'm getting at here is that by learning to use all of our other faculties without relying on the dominant one, sight, we actually perform even better than when we can see. By learning to do things without seeing we become more careful, patient, precise, exact, dexterous, and balanced in situations when we can see.

So for this training you are invited to expand your senses and intuition in a primal way by walking blindfolded in nature. This takes patience, guts, and the use of all your faculties and senses. It will also require you to move beyond what you perceive as your limitations and tap into feelings and intuitions that connect you on an energetic level with your surroundings. This happens when you let the person you think you are fall away so as to open up to the reality that exists beyond the confines of thought, intellect, and sight.

For this training you will need a partner to lead you safely. You and your partner should take turns being the participant and the leader; you will both be co-creating these experiences. Your partner will be walking in front of you as your guide because you will be blindfolded. First, locate a place in nature suitable for this training. You can start out in an open space or on a trail that is relatively flat and doesn't have too many obstructions such as fallen trees, rocks, or roots. Once you get more proficient at this you can do this anywhere. Grab a bandana or scarf for a blindfold and arrive at your destination.

+ Perform a good AT session of standard formulas mixed with visualization formulas of walking the trail without sight, along with affirmation formulas to boost your momentum.

---

*When making black-and-white prints, a dim red bulb is used, but when developing negatives the room must be absolutely lightless; any light whatsoever will ruin the film.

+ When ready, take a position one arm length in back of your guide and put on your blindfold.

+ Lightly place one of your hands on the leader's shoulder so you can follow behind at arm's length. Do not lean on your partner like a crutch. As the partner leading starts to walk, you follow behind by gently resting your hand on her shoulder. There is no verbal communication during this training unless absolutely necessary.

+ At this point simply get accustomed to the format of silently walking in tandem— the rhythm of it, and walking without sight. On easy ground most people get used to this quickly.

+ When you are ready, move to a little more challenging terrain (but you will still want to be on some sort of a trail). On a trail with more features the leader's task becomes more detailed and important. For example, if crossing a fallen log (in the early stages of training this should be done only if the log is on the ground; later, with more experience, you can scramble over anything), the leader can slow or stop and tap her foot on the log so that you know it's there. As she crosses over the log you will notice the change in her body movement, and you will intuit from her movement what you should also do. Do not talk to each other! Another example could be embedded or loose stones on the ground. In this case the partner leading can tap on the stones or shuffle her feet across them. Whatever the case, you must feel and intuit from your partner and the trail what you are walking on or over.

+ The really enjoyable part of this training is when you become comfortable doing this and working as a team, at which point your partner will slowly transform into just another feature of the environment. When this happens you will experience all the nuances of the trail, and without your sense of sight your other senses will expand. You will hear more (birds chirping, quaking leaves, babbling brook, etc.); you will feel more (sunlight and shade, breezes, warmer or cooler spots); and smells you don't normally notice will become much more apparent.

+ When you have become confident enough you can let go of the leader's shoulder. At this point the leader's job is essentially the same, but now you are not actually touching someone ahead of you and have lost that sense of her body motion, especially with regard to obstacles. The leading partner will continue tapping on obstacles or shuffling feet on loose rock, and if there are no obstacles the leader must be creative so you can follow behind. For example, if you are walking on grass or soil the leader may have to stamp a little harder on the ground so you can hear her. Now that you are not in physical contact with the leader you must heighten your sound awareness and intuition. Do not throw your arms up in front of you; this will do nothing but distract you. Your partner is there and won't let anything happen to you. Relax and embrace the darkness; become one with it. Allow your senses to expand and have fun.

Comments and considerations: As you might notice, this primal-mind training is also an exercise of attention for the partner who is leading. It is a good idea to switch places so as to learn both aspects of this training and therefore absorb even more. Another thing: working with the same partner(s) on an ongoing basis for these kinds of partner trainings will invariably produce the best results. As your confidence level increases you can tackle more and more difficult terrain, and your attention to what you feel will grow, and you'll start to trust your feelings about your surroundings at a level close to the trust you have in your sight. This is not only significant on a physical and practical level, it also serves as a reflection of how you see yourself and your life. When you give yourself an opportunity to work without the use of your sight you are embracing the unknown, the mystery. You are sending a clear message to yourself and to the world that you are not afraid of the unknown and in fact you are willing to face it head-on. This is an attitude that may be completely foreign to you. It is an attitude of strength, courage, and ultimately one of self-empowerment. The mysteries of life are the same in the dark as in the light, and sometimes we see more not after we take the blindfold off, but when we put it on.

Training #36
The Magic of Water

If one would have to choose a short list of things on planet Earth that could be classified as miracles, surely water would have to be at the top of the list. Nevertheless, people in Western cultures rarely think about water unless for whatever reason we don't have it. We simply turn on the faucet and flush the toilet without giving it any further thought. I'm not going to preach here about environmental ethics, but in terms of primal-mind awareness it is relevant to acknowledge that most of us don't know where the water in our pipes comes from or where our toilet water goes. If your local water authority or water commission has an open house of its facilities, going on such a tour can be a fascinating and eye-opening experience.

Most of us here in the United States don't give the availability of clean water a second thought. However, in parts of the country this is becoming a serious issue. As of this writing (the beginning of 2015) there are seven states running out of water. Exceptional drought is the worst, followed by extreme drought and severe drought. The following statistics come from the U.S. Drought Monitor, as reported by the U.S. Department of Agriculture, the National Oceanic and Atmospheric Administration (NOAA), and the National Drought Mitigation Center at the University of Nebraska, Lincoln.

Texas: severe drought 56.1 percent; extreme drought 39.9 percent (fourth highest in the country); exceptional drought 20.7 percent (third highest). Much of north and central Texas, including all of the Texas Panhandle, is covered in exceptional drought. The drought is having a large impact on the state's agriculture.

Oklahoma: severe drought 64.5 percent; extreme drought 50.1 percent (second highest); exceptional drought 30.4 percent (highest in the country). Severe drought covers over half of Oklahoma, up from roughly 33 percent one year ago. In March, the Oklahoma Emergency Drought Relief Commission awarded more than $1 million to several drought-ridden communities in the state.

Arizona: severe drought 76.3 percent; extreme drought 7.7 percent (ninth highest); exceptional drought 0.0 percent. Unlike other states suffering the most from drought, no part of Arizona experienced exceptional drought. Severe drought conditions, however, engulf more than three-quarters of the state.

Kansas: severe drought 80.8 percent; extreme drought 48.1 percent (third highest); exceptional drought 2.8 percent (sixth highest). Like several states running out of water, 80 percent of Kansas is engulfed in at least severe drought, an increase from one year ago when roughly 70 percent of the state was in severe drought.

New Mexico: severe drought 86.2 percent; extreme drought 33.3 percent (sixth highest); exceptional drought 4.5 percent (fifth highest). More than 86 percent of New Mexico is in severe drought, more than any state except Nevada and California. Additionally, one-third of the state is in extreme drought.

Nevada: severe drought 87.0 percent; extreme drought 38.7 percent (fifth highest); exceptional drought 8.2 percent (fourth highest). Nearly 40 percent of Nevada is in extreme drought, among the highest rates in the country. According to the Las Vegas Valley Water District, the main cause of drought has been below-average snowfall in the Rocky Mountains. Melting snow from the Rockies eventually makes its way into Lake Mead, which provides most of the Las Vegas Valley with water. John Entsminger, head of both the LVVWD and the Southern Nevada Water Authority, said that the effects of drought on the state have been "every bit as serious as a Hurricane Katrina or a Superstorm Sandy."[5]

California: severe drought 100.0 percent; extreme drought 76.7 percent (highest in the country); exceptional drought 24.8 percent (second highest). California is experiencing the worst drought conditions in the country, with more than 76 percent of the state in extreme drought. Drought in California has worsened considerably in recent years. Severe drought conditions cover the entire state, and the governor of California has declared a state of emergency. The shortage of potable water has been so severe that California is now investing in long-term solutions like desalination plants.

Here are some more facts about water from the U.S. Environmental Protection Agency and the U.S. Geological Survey[6]:

- Water covers about 71 percent of the earth's surface.
- Only 2.5 percent of the earth's water is freshwater, while 97.5 percent is saltwater.
- Only a little more than 1.2 percent of all freshwater is surface water found in lakes, rivers, streams, ponds, and swamps, which serve most of life's needs.
- 30.1 percent of the earth's freshwater is groundwater (in the ground).
- 68.7 percent of the earth's freshwater is trapped in glaciers.
- A ten-meter rise in sea levels due to melting glaciers would flood 25 percent of the population of the United States.
- There is more freshwater in the earth's atmosphere than in all of the rivers on the planet combined. If all of the water vapor in the atmosphere fell at once, distributed evenly, it would only cover the earth with about an inch of water.
- In the United States in 2010, we used about 275 billion gallons of surface water per day and about 79.3 billion gallons of groundwater per day.
- Nearly one-half of the water used by Americans is used for thermoelectric power generation.
- In one year, the average American residence uses over 100,000 gallons (indoors and outside).
- Individual Americans use about 100 gallons of water per day.
- At fifty gallons a day, residential Europeans use about half the water that residential Americans use.

UNESCO currently estimates that 783 million people do not have access to clean water, and almost 2.5 billion people do not have access to adequate sanitation.[7] Many people in the scientific and intelligence communities believe that in the future there is a high probability that wars will be fought over water, eclipsing current wars over religion and oil. In a 2012 report, the U.S. director of national intelligence warned that lack of access to water—as in India and other countries—was a source of conflict that could potentially compromise U.S. national security.[8]

Here in the United States it goes without saying that we need to stop overusing this precious resource. On a primal level we can cultivate a closer relationship with water by taking note of its subtler qualities. Many primal cultures I have lived among, including the Huichol of Western Mexico, are so connected to their bodies of water that they name them (not like a place, but like a person) and even make pilgrimages to them. The fundamental energy of water is one that anyone can feel and connect to when doing so with an open mind and heart. This should come as no surprise when we consider that we humans are anywhere from 55 to 78 percent water by weight.

Two amazing qualities of water make it a completely unique form of matter. Matter, of course, is all around us; it's the air you breathe, the book you are reading. Matter is the stuff you touch and see. Matter is defined as anything that has mass and takes up space. Matter is found in three major forms, solid, liquid, and gas, and water is the only form of matter on Earth that can be found naturally in all three states. The other distinct feature of water is that it is a universal solvent—more substances dissolve in water than in any other liquid, including sulfuric acid.

The structure and essence of water allows it to metamorphose into different states as its three-dimensional microstructures form and dissolve millions of times a second. When water flows, it carries, picks up, and distributes information as it responds and changes within its environment. For example, if we pour water through our hands, the water dissolves and picks up physical elements on our skin as well as the vibratory pulse of our being. The water is thus changed; it now contains a part of us. And it will change again as soon as it touches something else. The same can be said for us. When we are submerged in a natural body of water, the water transmits physical and vibrational information to our human organism. We are affected by the numerous unique qualities of the water—its flow and temperature, its nutrients (minerals and salts), as well as the particular feeling and energy being exuded by its fluid body. We are changed—we have now become part of the water until we leave the water and are then affected by something else.

Moreover, for both the water and for us, the story doesn't end here because we both have a memory. Water affects and is affected by everything that it meets, and it carries both a physical and a vibrational memory of its encounter with us. This may be at a very subtle level, but it will carry it just the same—just as we carry the memory of the water within us on different levels. This is one of the core reasons we work with water at a primal level. Once we become water we are never the same, and the more experiences we have with the myriad personalities of water, and the deeper we dive in to these experiences, the more we learn as a result of placing ourselves directly into a natural form of wisdom that contains the energy and vibrations of both the earth and the cosmos.

Water appears in different forms, each with its own qualities and feelings (see table 13.1 on page 207).

Here is a sample AT-PM exercise to connect with water at a psycho-physiological level:

+ Find a body of water such as a river, pond, stream, lake, or the ocean. Approach the water and assess its physical and subtle characteristics. Is it calm or raging, shallow or deep? Does it appear safe to enter, are there rocks or boulders visible, how does it smell? Sit or stand quietly next to the water, and soak up the unique qualities being exuded by the water, and listen to its unique song.
+ Use your mind to compare your emotional state to that of the water; relate the qualities of this body of water to specific past experiences where your emotional being mirrored the feeling of this body of water.

✦ Relate to the water at a physical level by using your bodily memory of times past to remember physical experiences that share similar qualities with this body of water; for example, times when your body felt calm, or flowing, or raging.

✦ Contemplate the environmental situation of this body of water. Where did it come from, and where is it headed? What are the physical threats you can see or otherwise know about that jeopardize the health of this water? Is there anything you can see, determine, or know about that actively protects this body? What do you notice about the overall health of this body?

✦ Touch the water, and notice how the interconnectedness of the whole body means that by touching one area of water you affected the whole body of water at a subtle but real level. At the same time realize and feel that the touch of the water has subtly affected your own entire organism as well.

✦ Now sit close to the water and use a combination of AT and PM formulas to get ready to enter the water.

✦ Begin with two minutes of passive breathing, silently repeating *I breathe me.*

✦ Passively focus on each of the areas below, one at a time.

✦ Starting with your dominant arm, silently repeat three times *My right* (or *left*) *arm is heavy.*

✦ Here inject your own formula related to physical connection (e.g., *I hear the song of this . . .* [*stream, river, pond, lake,* or *ocean*]). Silently repeat it six times.

✦ Silently repeat three times *My heartbeat is calm and strong.*

✦ Here inject your own formula related to your physical connection to the water (e.g., *I can smell and taste the unique qualities of this . . .*). Silently repeat it six times.

✦ Silently repeat three times *My solar plexus is warm.*

✦ Here inject your own formula related to your mental connection with the water (e.g., *My body is 60 percent water; I need water to survive*). Silently repeat it six times.

✦ Silently repeat three times *My arms and legs are warm.*

✦ Here inject your own formula related to your emotional connection with the water (this formula will really depend on the form of the water you are sitting by, e.g., *The pond reflects my calm emotional state*). Silently repeat this six times.

✦ Silently repeat six times *My neck and back are warm.*

TABLE 13.1. QUALITIES OF WATER

Water Form	Qualities
Stream	Delicate flow, winding fluid motion, graceful or dainty song, shallow depth, clear appearance, light and youthful wisdom, creative, joyful
River	Mixing of calm near shore and powerful and even dangerous currents in the middle, potential for soft or roaring song, hidden knowledge and mysteries, longer and deeper memory, more extensive experience
Pond	Calm, reflective, soothing, nurturing, safe yet mysterious
Lake	Expansive, filled with hidden power, capable of displaying many emotions, support for many forms of life
Ocean	Awesome, very approachable and knowable at a shallow level but also deeply secretive, incomprehensibly diverse in the amount of life it supports, vast, ultimately powerful

✦ While still aware of the warmth in your neck and back, say to yourself *I am very quiet.*

✦ Remain relaxed for a minute or two.

✦ Cancel.

✦ Repeat this sequence two more times.

✦ After your last cancel, and if safe to do so, enter the water and open yourself to the total experience of now being a part of the body of water. Feel the vibration of the water's body influence your own water body. Be aware of how your movements and vibrations affect the body of water. Listen, smell, and taste the unique qualities of the water. Fill your mind with the water. Let the water infuse your organism with its unique memory and luminous energy. Absorb and reflect the water with your whole human organism. Stay at least a half hour in the water unless it is unbearably cold; a total of two to four hours spent in and near the body of water is best. If you have a calm body of water to work with you can use a raft or canoe to alternately get into the water and float on the water. To truly gather a deep feeling of a particular body of water requires many visits throughout the different seasons of the year; nevertheless, even one significant encounter with a body of water can provide incalculable benefit and self-knowledge.

Training #37
Primal Fire Connection

Mastery of fire is one of the most significant milestones of the human race. With the ability to make and control fire our species was able to spread out across the globe, even to the most inhospitable places. For our hunter-gatherer forebears fire was probably the most useful and magical force they could possibly dream of. Fire provided warmth and protection. Thanks to fire's ability to cook food and smoke meat, our ancestors were able to make the meat of the animals they hunted more digestible and palatable and could cook plants to eat that were otherwise inedible, thereby reducing the chance of starvation. Fire made our primal ancestors more efficient in other ways too. With torches they could remain active and productive after dark. This helped shape complex social behavior, as it allowed families and communities to gather together. As the control of fire became more refined, such as by blowing the flame through pipes of reed, the people created bowls, cradles, and canoes out of wood. Eventually humans learned to efficiently cultivate crops and subjugate animals, but even then fire was still a central element of daily life, as most simple homes contained a hearth or fireplace, while the homes of the rich and the palaces of rulers contained movable stoves and central furnaces that provided heat for several rooms at a time. The use of fire was also essential to the development of pottery and, later, metalworking.

At this point in our long history with this element there came a significant change in our relationship with fire. We became more demanding of it; instead of simply trying to control it and move it around to serve our needs, we felt the need to significantly intensify it in the name of "progress." The development of the blast furnace to liquefy metal would eventually lead to the Industrial Revolution. To this day, fire still forms a central part of our technological existence. Unfortunately we are now using fire in a completely unsustainable way. Not too long ago we humans broke the natural cycles that keep the earth alive as a result of our extraction and burning of what we humans call *fossil fuels*, which in reality are anaerobically decomposed and buried dead organisms of eons past that have no natural business being on the earth's surface. Western civilization is now completely dependent on fossil fuels for industry and transportation. Drilling under the earth and sea could easily be seen as one of the worst decisions our species has ever made.

This book is not the place to go into detailing the vast number of tragedies that have resulted in just the last century from this one human activity. The point I want to make here is that on the most primal level the pathological actions of humans are in many ways related to the loss of awareness of the sacredness of fire that our primal ancestors once had. Fire offers a way to alter our consciousness when we cross the threshold of knowing that a healthy relationship with the fundamental energy of fire can lead to a healthy relationship with the world, and also with our individual human organism.

In the following training we're going to incorporate many significant techniques that I have learned from various primal cultures that still exist today. However, as I have said in all my previous books, and I'll say again here, it is not enough to simply copy primal peoples to gain primal knowledge. We are people living in the modern world; therefore our techniques of personal growth have to be applicable and available for use in our lives as modern people. This means taking our cues from primal people and then adapting them for use in our world. In terms of fire, this means expanding our view of fire to something more than just the extraction of fuel to power our automobiles or the few moments we might spend creating a cozy or romantic atmosphere with a candle, fireplace, or campfire. In this training we will experience the four aspects of the element of fire: connection, protection, purification, and intention.

Let's start with connection. Connecting to fire might seem like a romantic or even silly activity to many people. And if you don't get it right away that is perfectly understandable. It actually took me many years. I can't tell you how many times I participated in the rituals and ceremonies of primal peoples where the sacred fire was the main component, and I truly felt like an outsider looking in. Now, I am one of those people who has always loved making and being around a fire, but actually connecting to fire was beyond my scope of comprehension. Eventually I learned through experience to shift and expand my perception, simply because at a primal level we can all feel the energy of fire. This is because fire is so easy for us to connect to. This can be observed in the way we now have a fireplace that doesn't actually function as a primary source of heat, whether in a home, restaurant, or lodge, but rather is there because people enjoy the conscious and subconscious presence of fire.

The most time-tested primal tool of protection is the sacred fire, especially at night. When we invite the energy of fire by igniting it in the center of our activity we come under the metaphysical protection of this element. The psychophysiology and physics of this are not understandable within our current paradigm of science, so how this happens is really not explainable, but it is certainly quantifiable. I have seen it happen so many times that for me it is a situation as real as a dog protecting its master from a stranger in the night.

This leads us to the purification and intentions we can invoke by working with fire. These two primal situations will be the basis for this training. But first I'm going to introduce you to a primal manner in which to bring fire alive and keep it going in a special way.

How you actually ignite your fire is not that important for this training. It's not my intention to teach you how to make fire by rubbing two sticks together or any other primitive fire-making techniques. A simple match or lighter will do. The important thing here is not ignition but structure. The structure of the fire is important because we want to intentionally make this fire special so we can interact with it in unconventional ways. The technique I will now share with you is born from my experiences with the Huichol (Wirrarika) people. If you truly don't have access to a place where you can have a fire, then a candle can be used, but you will miss some very important actions and energy exchanges. Nevertheless, if using a candle I suggest you still read the following section.

+ The first thing to do is clear a small area where the fire will be. We will not be making a huge bonfire, just one big enough to bring forth the flowing flames and numinous qualities we can connect with.
+ Collect or bring with you enough fist-size (or maybe a little bigger) rocks to place in a circle on the ground, inside which you will make your fire. This is referred to as the *bed*.
+ Inside the bed place the "pillow," which is a fairly hefty log, six to twelve inches in diameter and long enough to span your rock circle. Typically it is placed in the east. But if you are going on a trip or pilgrimage or want to connect to certain place, the pillow can be placed in that direction. However, east is the default direction for the rising sun.
+ The actual fuel (food) for the fire consists of small-diameter sticks (no bigger than wrist size) that are placed all in one direction. This is accomplished by resting the tips of the sticks (called *arrows*) one at a time on the pillow, in such a way that one end of the stick lies on the pillow, and the other end of the stick rests on the ground inside the circle of stones. In this way all the sticks point in one direction. For those of you accustomed to making a campfire to cook food this might seem odd. The most efficient way to make a hot fire for cooking is to lay sticks in a crisscross fashion to allow copious amounts of oxygen to flow between the sticks. But this is not a cook fire. Here our arrows signify a single-minded intention: to connect with fire. We don't place our sticks willy-nilly or in opposing directions because this opposes our intention. By intentionally and carefully placing our arrows in one direction we focus our attention on making our fire in a special way.
+ Once you have cleared a small area, made a ring of rocks, and set up a pillow and your first arrows, you can use various things to get the fire going. The thin, dead lower branches from a pine or other resinous tree are perfect, but any natural, thin, dry material such as dry grass will work. Sometimes when I go to an unfamiliar place I will carry with me a small amount of natural

fire-starter material. This is usually made of sawdust that has been compressed into small bars. They are easy to find in camping supply stores or hardware stores. Whatever you need to use is okay, just avoid using fossil fuels like gas, diesel, or lighter fluid.

✦ Make sure you have a good quantity of sticks set aside to be used as arrows to place on the fire as it burns. Ideally these are fairly straight sticks that are equal to or thinner than the diameter of your wrist. To keep the fire alive you will be constantly feeding it arrows throughout this activity.

✦ When all is prepared, light your fire and open yourself to the flowing flames, heat, and smell of the fire. From now on it is important to make a personal connection to the fire. The most potent way I have found to do this is the same way many tribal peoples make this kind of connection, and that is to now refer to the fire as Grandfather Fire. Most (if not all) tribal cultures consider fire to be a masculine element. Of course, there are female energies and elements as well. The Huichol call the energy that animates life Grandmother Growth, and all forms of water are referred to as mothers and given a specific name. In any case the idea is to personify the fire, so we speak to it as we would a close friend or relative or a distinguished and respected grandfather. But think of Grandfather Fire as more of an archetype than an actual person.

Whether doing this training with groups or individuals there are always five energetic stages to complete while working with Grandfather Fire. I like to explain these as doorways or gates that one passes through. Each successive gate leads to an area of increased clarity and intention. When experiencing this training in a group setting, the participants take turns until the gate is complete, and then the whole group moves on to the next gate, taking turns once again.

The First Gate

What we are trying to do in the first gate is to open the energetic door with fire through communication, and there is nothing that we know better than our own story. If you are doing this training in a group setting it is important that everyone make a sacred agreement that nothing said around the circle of fire ever leaves without permission. The only task of those who are not speaking is to listen in a nonjudgmental way to the person speaking and to feed him or her with good thoughts and intentions. In this respect these thoughts and intentions become for the speaker the extended body of the fire at the center of the circle. In this first gate you will tell the story of your past to Grandfather Fire. In terms of time this is usually the longest and yet the least difficult gate. For this first gate and the other four to come start out by stating out loudly, "Grandfather Fire, in front of you and all my companions [even if you are alone in this ritual you are not really ever alone in nature] I would like to share with you . . . [here inject some important parts of your personal history; e.g., plans for the future]."

From now until the end of this training you will be speaking out loud to Grandfather Fire. We as humans have been given this remarkable capacity for speech, and it is the best way of moving and expressing energy. If you do this training silently or telepathically it will lose 90 percent or more of its effectiveness. So tell Grandfather the story of your life with feeling and emotion. Be aware not to fall into the trap of making this merely a resume of factual statements. So instead of saying something like, "then I did this and then I did that," make it more like, "I (did whatever) because . . ." and "as a result I . . . "

Try to keep your words flowing. This means you should avoid stopping to think. On the contrary, this should be one continuous stream of words and energy flowing from you and going into Grandfather Fire. You don't have to be specifically chronological or even make sense; you could even talk gibberish, as long as you do it with feeling and heart. Talk about different phases of your life, friends, places where you lived, loved ones, school, careers, special places, romances, good times, bad times, whatever. Take as much time as you need. When you really get into this it's not unusual to actually remember events in your life that you have long forgotten.

The Second Gate

This gate typically is the most difficult of the five. It's called the *energetic confession*. In this case we are not talking about the kind of confession made in a church with the intention of being absolved from some sort of sin. This type of confession is purely about energy, not morals. It in no way concerns how anyone else might view your actions. The reason you are energetically confessing is not because you may have done something wrong in the eyes of another person or an institution but rather because the events you are confessing have left an energetic stain on your true being, and this is the chance to invite the purifying qualities of the fire to help burn them away.

For example, many times it is hard for people to truly say good-bye to a relative, friend, or past lover, so they carry this unresolved issue around with them for the rest of their lives. In this moment with the fire you would say that good-bye. You would use the person's name and talk to the fire just as if that person *is* the fire. Another common energetic stain is not saying thank you to someone who has helped you. Now is that time. Use names. Bring out the emotions behind the event. Maybe you smoke or drink or have a drug habit you're having a hard time letting go of. These are energetic stains, not sins. Give them to the fire. You could be feeling guilty or ashamed about something. Or maybe you made a promise you didn't keep, either to yourself or someone else. You probably get the idea by now. The main thing is to not hold anything back. If you don't let go of whatever it is, it becomes an energetic ball and chain. By releasing the weight you have been tethered to, you allow yourself to soar.

The Third Gate

In this stage you talk to the fire about your present life. This happens in the same way as before, in one continuous flow of words from you to Grandfather Fire. Usually, but not always, this gate is easier than the previous one. Simply talk to Grandfather about what is going on in your life, be it positive or not so positive. Be specific and honest. As before, give specific names and reveal your true feelings and emotions. Again, avoid giving a resume; speak from your heart.

The Fourth Gate

Talk to Grandfather Fire about how you feel *right now*, sitting next to him as you talk to him. Tell him how you got to this moment, why you are here, what you hope to achieve. How's the weather? How does your body feel? Don't hold back, be in the here and now and tell Grandfather all about it.

The Fifth Gate

This is the gate of the hypothetical future. This future doesn't come about by wishing or praying; it manifests by *doing*. Tell Grandfather what you want. Spell it all out, and most importantly, tell him how you are going to get there. Be specific. Avoid statements like, "I want to save the world" or "I want to end hunger." Sure, maybe you do, but to accomplish anything in life we have to make our goals specific. If I say, "I want to write a new book," that's great, but I need to add something like, "and I'm going to start writing my new book on Saturday and have my outline done within two weeks." The point is to state attainable goals for the future, and then back them up by telling the fire specifically what you're going to do to attain them.

Now that you have passed through this primal training, the element of fire can always be there for you, in your darkest moments as well as your triumphs. Oftentimes when I need energy or encouragement I visualize a meeting with the fire I had in a specific place. Other times I simply use a candle to connect. Through a candle you can feed the fire daily with your thoughts, problems, feelings, emotions, inspirations, goals, etc. Grandfather Fire does not judge and can be a powerful resource of numinous intelligence in your life.

14
Going Deeper into Primal Rites of Passage in Nature

In the scheme of trainings for the renewal and development of primal mind, a more advanced technique is the vision quest. This is a rite of passage that was and in some cases still is one of the most important rituals of tribal peoples of North America. In the last thirty years or so the vision quest has increasingly gained in popularity among nonnative spiritual seekers around the Western world. In terms of primal mind it is an experience of transformation and awareness that I hope everyone experiencing the trainings in this book will try.

In the days before such medicine plants as peyote, mushrooms, and datura became popular as a means of accessing visions, the tribal peoples of North America relied on induced suffering and hardship in the wilderness to summon up the visionary spirits that would teach them how to live. A young person would travel alone to a remote area where his people knew that the spirits of nature were strong and lively. This could be a dense forest, a mountaintop, a swamp, or any other remote area where the powers dwelled. In this place the young person would stay for several days and nights, fasting from both food and water, wearing nothing but a loincloth, to endure whatever Mother Nature and the spirits had in store. In solitude and outside the sphere of village life, the initiate sat silent and alone, fasting, naked to the elements, open to receive anything that would stimulate the mind, body, and spirit. Stripped of clothing, material possessions, and the protection of family and tribe, the initiate was forced to learn about and dive deep into his or her own physical and psychic resources to deal with the perils posed by wild animals, storms, hunger, thirst, and boredom. In this state the person was completely free of the normal social concerns of everyday life. Little by little, as the initiate became increasingly empty of human-centered wants and thoughts, the hidden abilities of the psyche would arise and the consciousness of the initiate would expand to perceive that consciousness is all around. When this happened, visions would come.

Visions acquired in this manner must not be confused or relegated to internal processes of the mind alone, because what is happening here is an expansion of consciousness whereby the items and energies of the world that are normally seen as external to the human organism are now viewed as part of a continuum that includes both what is internal and external to the initiate. In other words, there is no inside or outside of the head or mind. Both of these realities meet and are bound together by what can loosely be called consciousness. In this visionary state there is little or no perceived separation between different types of living beings. Plants wave and acknowledge the vision quester, while animals and insects and birds deliver messages. In this visionary state the lines of nonverbal communication are open, and a dialog between the human organism and the other species in the environment begins; the possibilities of this kind of communication become limitless.

For adults in modern culture, where everything humanly possible is done to avoid the kind of hardships entailed in this rite of passage, the decision to embark on a quest for a vision is one that is usually brought on by some sort of life crisis, something serious enough to test one's inner strength and determination in such a way that healing becomes the only solution. Normally when people need help they automatically turn to a counselor, minister, psychiatrist, medium, doctor, or family and friends. But in this case the person must realize deep down that the only way to be healed is to heal oneself. The only way to truly go forward is to leave everything behind and scale the mountain of fears and dreams without someone else holding a safety line.

For many people the decision to embark on such a quest is a truly heroic act because it signifies a departure from the pitiful dependence of believing someone else will solve our problems. Many people whom I have worked with in this type of rite, as well as other intense rites of passage, have valiantly owned up to their specific life circumstances and have taken responsibility for making a better life for themselves. Some have been victims of violence, abuse, or rape. Others have battled depression from loss of a loved one, a miscarriage or an abortion or are in a life-and-death struggle with substance or alcohol abuse. But many others come to the vision quest as a result of purely wanting to find meaning in their lives. Even outwardly successful people living the cliché of the American Dream oftentimes lack the inner resources and inner spiritual development so common to indigenous peoples, for whom these kinds of rites of passage provide guidance that comes from a much bigger source of mystery and power than the world of purely human concerns. And so we find that increasingly the successful businessperson, as well as the mother of happy and grown children, comes to the solitude of the vision quest to seek answers for the biggest of questions.

There are basically two ways to enter this experience—go it alone or seek out an experienced person or organization that facilitates these kinds of quests. For those of you wanting to try going it alone I'm going to provide you with a format to do so. There are also many books available that can be helpful. My favorite, which I highly recommend, is *The Book of the Vision Quest: Personal Transformation in the Wilderness,* by Steven Foster. This book is special because not only does it eloquently explain the vision quest, it also includes comments and stories from dozens of vision questers who have participated in Steven's School of Lost Borders programs. Steven passed away in 2003, but his legacy and school live on.

However you go about it, the truth all boils down to the fact that what you will receive in any rite of passage, initiation, ritual, ceremony, or offering will be directly proportional to what you put into it. In this case, there is absolutely no way that talking, intellectualizing, theorizing, or any attempt at influencing by means of our ordinary ways of manipulation will have any effect on the level of transformation you will receive during the vision quest. The vision you will attain during this journey of primal connection to the spirits of nature and the flowing consciousness of the cosmos is truly ineffable. Only by laying yourself bare, emptying yourself through fasting and solitude, and recounting your problems to a mountain or a spider that is crawling up your leg, will you make yourself small and humble and thus open to receive the vision that will be reflected back to you by the mirror of nature.

There are no shortcuts or magical formulas in these kinds of rites, because each person brings with himself his own unique story, needs, and wants. A framework for the rite is provided to give it a time-tested ritual structure that has proven to be helpful in drawing out the person's inner perceptions. But aside from this general framework, the rite becomes alive purely as a result of the interaction between the person and the environment, and the melding of the two. In the vision quest nobody will be there to give you opinions or impose their influence on you. Your counselor is the wind, your supporter the earth, your nourishment the sun, and your only companions are the wild animals. In this sense you will transform yourself into one of your ancient ancestors who lived in a wild and untamed world free of cell phone towers, 24-hour television, and high-speed Internet.

Training #38
Primal Mind and the Quest for Vision*

The first stage of the vision quest is the departure. In this stage you remove yourself from your everyday life and leave behind your family, friends, job, and responsibilities both at the physical and psychological level. When you depart on the vision quest journey you will never come

---

*Portions of this training are excerpted from the author's *Ecoshamanism*.

back to the same place from where you left. In this sense, with your very first step you leave your old self behind and begin walking into your new state of being. You depart from your ordinary life and cross the border into the unknown. Sometimes it is helpful to associate this crossing with the symbolism of a doorway, threshold, gate, or passageway. There is a crack between the worlds into which you humbly pass through. Again, there is no magical formula for making this entrance; it is purely a matter of consciousness. Similarly to how you can't force yourself to go to sleep but rather sleep takes you and shifts your state of consciousness, so it is with the departure in the vision quest. It is like moving through the paradox of a "gateless gate."

When you have gone into this crack between the worlds of consciousness and through the gateless gate you arrive in a new land. This is the actual experience of the vision quest as you arrive at a chosen place in the wilderness where you will stay fasting for at least three nights. This is a sacred place far removed from human civilization. In this natural setting many things will happen to you. It is vitally important to enter into a respectful relationship with the place from the very first moment you arrive.

The first thing you must do is explain to the land what you are doing and make a gesture of offering to the place. The most powerful way to do this is with your own blood. This can be simply done by making a small hole in the ground with your bare hands while talking to the land about what you are doing there. Then prick your finger with a needle and while placing a few drops in the hole tell the sacred place that your blood is your offering and that the union of your blood with the soil symbolizes your desire and intention of becoming one with the land. Watch as the earth absorbs your blood, and then cover the hole. If you light a fire in the night it is good to place the fire on this offering.

During your stay in this sacred place countless things will happen, and it is impossible to say what they might include. It is common to initially experience periods of intense questioning as to your motives for being alone in the wilderness, fear that maybe you are simply going nuts, denial of the reasons you are doing it, depression, or feelings of intense self-pity. This is completely normal and is just one of the stages that a person of the modern world must pass through in order to become one again with the land and the cosmos. Until you are emptied and freed from these heavy and constricting thoughts and emotions, you won't be able to soar. One of the key reasons this rite of passage places you completely alone and fasting in the wilderness is to bring these feelings out and lay them bare before the spirits of nature.

During the three-night vision quest it has been my experience that in contrast to what my rational mind is expecting to receive or would consider to be a really huge happening, it is more common to experience many unexpected insights or visions from completely unforeseen sources. For example, on my very first vision quest I can remember that instead of seeing or talking to some sort of wise old spirit being, which would have been congruent with what I expected or wished would happen, I spent most of the first two days dealing with swarms of both flies and mosquitoes. During that time it seemed like the big deal of my vision quest had been reduced to simply placing myself in a position of being tortured by these aggressively savage little beasts, and I was more than a little perturbed at both the insects and myself for being there. But what eventually happened made the whole ordeal worthwhile. The flies and mosquitoes gave me exactly what I needed in that moment: they pushed my patience and my will to the absolute breaking point. Their bombardment of me was so intense that I freaked out not once, but so many times that I became physically and mentally exhausted. The resulting shift in consciousness forced me to view the world in a way I had never experienced before. Seeing the world with new eyes is one of the most valuable benefits of the vision quest, and on that day I went from seeing those irritating insects as nothing more than swarms of troublesome and annoying pests to acknowledging them as divine messengers of the nature spirits. When I finally *saw* what was truly going on and stopped both my internal struggle and my outward battle with the insects and just sat there with a feeling of peace and resignation, the insects ceased to be a distraction and eventually a strong wind blew up and they were gone within an hour.

My vision was gratefully earned, and I was magically transformed from a person easily irritated by trivialities into someone who peacefully receives and acknowledges the gifts of life, which was a completely foreign state of mind to me at that time in my life. The insects delivered this vision and transformation in the most effective way possible. In this sense I was visited by the nature spirits, just not in any form that my mind would have anticipated. The outcome of my ordeal with the flies and mosquitoes was that it affected me deeply enough that I was subsequently able to physically and psychically apply the lesson I learned to my everyday life and dealings with people, both on an intentional and on a subconscious level. After my first vision quest many people who knew me well commented on the change in the way I was able to handle stressful or potentially annoying situations with much more ease and with a kind of peaceful serenity. And not only did that experience affect my everyday life, it also raised my level of experience of other facets of my spiritual life.

For example, on my next vision quest it became quite clear after just a few moments in my spot, which was on the other side of the country in completely different terrain than the first time, my initial spirit helpers this time would be spiders. During those three days I met hundreds of spiders of many different species, and because of my previous experience with the flies and mosquitoes this time I was able right from the start to make peace with the spiders and just let them walk right over me, under me, on top of me, and even inside my clothes and blanket. Through the powerful agents of fasting and solitude, coupled with my peaceful attitude of openness and willingness to receive without preconceived judgments, I was able to have remarkable and enlightening conversations with many different and very insightful spiders. The spirits of that place had chosen to speak to me through these incredibly interesting and unique creatures. And even though I thought I was as open as possible to receiving whatever came, I have to admit that at one point, after consciously realizing that the sheer number of spiders that were coming to me one by one could not be mere coincidence, I felt a peculiar kind of awe that was almost frightening in knowing that I was truly at the mercy of the nature spirits of those woods, and that they were really talking to me in a way I could actually understand.

With this type of experience comes a certain level of responsibility in that when you are fortunate enough to receive messages, insights, or visions from the spirits of the natural world, they cannot be ignored, even if what they are telling you isn't what you want to hear or the requests they make of you seem too difficult to accomplish. In a nutshell, if you are not prepared to accept and act on the vision that the spirits of nature may have in store for you, you probably want to reconsider entering into this rite of passage.

Another significant consideration in undertaking this rite of passage is that the nature spirits will be asking something, or many things, of you. This is a vitally important aspect of connecting in a primal encounter with the nature spirits that rule and animate the world. You better listen to everything they are saying, not just those things you want or need to hear because they almost always ask something of you in return for their knowledge. This means that when you return from the threshold of the vision quest and step squarely back into your everyday life you will have to accomplish the tasks given to you, no matter how difficult they may be, because if you don't you might not only lose your chance for learning what they are trying to teach you, you may suffer the consequences that come from being deceitful and selfish enough to ask but not give. This should not be construed as something like the threat of damnation resulting from sinful activity but rather as a sort of universal karmic response to your actions that will be directly proportional to the level of reality you attach to receiving from the spirits.

The following is the basic structure and practical considerations of the vision quest:

Prepare Yourself and Your Equipment

This training includes two to three days of fasting (water is permissible). If you are not accustomed to fasting you will probably find this a difficult experience not only because of the physiological responses of your body but also because of the disconnection to the regimented psychological schedule that regular feeding times provide. Because of this it is wise to familiarize yourself before the quest by intentionally skipping meals for a few weeks and by eating light foods such vegetables, fruits, rice, and fish, and skipping heavier foods like beef, nuts, dairy products, and oily or fried foods. It is also good to engage in rigorous physical activity outdoors and to simply pay attention to your physical and emotional needs and avoid intoxication by alcohol or drugs.

Only you can decide what is completely essential to take with you on your quest. This will largely depend on your level of comfort and familiarity with being outdoors for three whole days and nights. If you are new to spending time outdoors it is a good idea to make a few trial runs at sleeping out overnight in a forest area that is not far from civilization in order to gain confidence and increase your skills. (Training #34 is also a good place to start.) If you are questing under the tutelage of an experienced guide that person should be able to provide the list of basic gear specific to the terrain you will submerged in. Aside from suitable clothes and footwear for the season, a general list of items to consider bringing would include water, a blanket or sleeping bag, fire-starting supplies in a waterproof container, a knife, a ground cloth or rain tarp, writing materials, a flashlight, and a first-aid kit

The trick behind the whole concept of bringing gear into this type of minimalistic rite is to find the balance between what you truly need to bring and what you dare not bring. For example, by my third quest I felt confident enough to lay myself as bare as I could so I didn't bring anything except the clothes I was wearing, water, and one blanket for three nights in the mountains of Colorado in October. Needless to say I was extremely cold at night because I didn't even allow myself the company of the fire, but my profound connection to the rising sun in the morning would never have reached the same intensity if I hadn't been so cold. More recently I haven't felt the need to be quite as extreme, and now I always have the fire for many reasons, including warmth.

Choose Your Place and Prepare Your Safety Strategy

If the rite is not being led by an experienced guide you should scope out your spot ahead of time and make sure that someone responsible knows exactly where you will be. You can even devise a check-up system whereby you and your supporter leave each other a signal at a predetermined spot close to your questing area to indicate that you are okay at certain intervals, such as once a day at noon. Otherwise it is important not to interact with the person checking on you. The idea is to leave a sign (a note, a pile of rocks, etc.) at a predetermined place so your helper will know you are okay but you don't actually see or talk to him.

Embarking on the Quest

Once you have arrived at your questing area it is normal to have feelings of having to keep busy. Generally speaking, there are simply no required activities in this rite; in fact, quite the contrary, the lack of activity produces reflection and submersion in the action that is unfolding around you, and the deeper you can dive into that reality and out of your purely selfish concerns the more profound your resulting experience. Since being alone in the wilderness is the perfect time to add AT to your experience, do so. Beginner and novice questers are encouraged not to engage in comforting activities done simply to keep busy, such as reading, playing musical instruments, making crafts, or any other type of intentional distraction. Other than gathering firewood in an area very close to your spot during the day and performing AT-PM sessions, the only other activities I encourage would be those that connect you directly to the land and that happen spontaneously. These include face or body painting using materials from the land, tree climbing (just high enough to be off the ground), exposing your naked body to the wind, and talking to and listening to the nighttime fire.

Return, Slowly

Upon returning to your everyday life it is good to avoid going right back into the frantic pace of modern society and to avoid as much as possible the manipulating psychological warfare of media and especially violent movies and TV. Also, it is a good idea to intentionally avoid any situations that might make you susceptible to manipulative people because your guard will be down and your consciousness will be altered in a way that you might not recognize potentially harmful deceptions. In the best-case scenario, give yourself a few days of transition between your wilderness vision quest and the urban jungle by staying somewhere halfway in between in order to better reflect on and digest your experience.

Fulfilling Your Vision and Commitments

If you have been blessed with insights and visions pertaining to your life, then you should begin whatever steps necessary to living congruently with your vision. Any offerings you made to the spirits of the place in order to "pay" for your vision should be accomplished as soon as possible to insure the balance of a reciprocal and healthy relationship with the spirits.

AT and the Vision Quest

For close to twenty years I included the vision quest as an annual or semiannual part of my life. During that time period I had no knowledge of AT. Since my first encounter with the standard AT formulas I have found practicing and integrating AT into my vision quests to be indispensable. By combining the standard formulas with free-form formulas, as we have done with many other trainings in this book that combine AT and PM, it is possible and highly probable to acquire even more from a vision-quest experience.

My suggestions in doing so are as follows:

- Engage in sessions of standard formulas, visualization, meditation, and energy-tunnel formulas combined with free-form formulas at least three times a day, especially upon waking up and when night rolls in. Engaging in more than three is desirable and helpful.

- AT is extremely helpful in those moments when you are so bored you feel like you're going out of your mind, or when you are in deep stages of self-doubt as to what you are doing and why.
- There are certain moments during the vision quest when you should actually call out for a vision. Sometimes these moments are those just described, and other times you simply feel the call. Literally calling out with your voice is the old-school method and is very effective. But remember, you also now have experience with AT and it can be extremely effective as well.

Here are some examples of how to use AT during a vision quest:

+ Upon waking, while still on the ground lying on your back, engage in two minutes of passive breathing, silently repeating *I breathe me.*
+ Passively focus on each of the areas below, one at a time.
+ Starting with your dominant arm, silently repeat three times *My right* (or *left*) *arm is heavy.*
+ Here inject your own formula related to setting the mood of your vision quest (e.g., *I am peaceful and open*). Repeat this six times. These free-form formulas can be said silently to yourself or out loud (out loud moves more energy).
+ Silently or out loud repeat three times *My heartbeat is calm and strong.*
+ Here inject your own formula related to why you are here (e.g., *Today I will petition for my vision*). Silently or out loud repeat this six times.
+ Silently or out loud repeat three times *My solar plexus is warm.*
+ Here inject your own formula related to where you are (e.g., *I am one with everything in this place*). Silently or out loud repeat this six times. While going through these formulas place in your mind all the elements of nature around you.
+ Silently or out loud repeat three times *My arms and legs are warm.*
+ Here inject your own formula related to support (e.g., *I ask the help of all the living beings around me*). Silently or out loud repeat this six times.
+ Silently or out loud repeat three times *My neck and back are warm.*
+ While still aware of the warmth in your arms and legs, say to yourself silently or out loud *I am very quiet.*

✦ Remain relaxed for a minute or two.
✦ Cancel.
✦ Repeat this sequence at least two more times.

When seeking a vision or insight, say the free-form formulas out loud and in a strong voice. These sessions should be done standing or sitting.

✦ Engage in two minutes of passive breathing, silently repeating *I breathe me*.
✦ In the same way as the previous session pick at least five standard formulas and between them add your own free-form formulas. As always, begin with your dominant arm and end with a standard formula. Here is an example of a free-form progression added between the standard formulas when petitioning for a vision:

I am here for a vision.
I offer my time and energy to connect with nature.
I humbly suffer for my vision.
I call out to the nature spirits of this place to grant my vision.

Additional considerations: Remember what was discussed earlier— it's imperative that you realize that messages, insights, and visions will more than likely arrive to you in a way you are not expecting. As was the case with my anecdotes about flies and the spiders, you may not "see" any sort of supernatural vision (although you just might); it may be that you hear whispers from the trees, or you decipher the songs of birds, or you get a message from the flames of your fire, etc. The main thing is to enter the quest open to *all* possibilities and without any pre-conceived notions.

Again, if you are not working with an experienced guide it would be prudent not to choose a place for your quest that is extremely iso-lated or where you could easily become lost. As long as your spot is completely devoid of human activity, free from the sounds of the urban jungle and in a healthy ecological condition, it need not be so remote as to pose undue risk. The underlying spirit behind the quest is not to see how far you can escape into the wilderness, but to encounter it and become part of it.

The five basic steps I have outlined here are just the bare bones to get you started. From this structure your personal spirit will meld with the forces of nature to help you create your own authentic experience. In the final analysis it will be your own tears and laughter, hardships and triumphs, intuition and spirit that will ultimately be your most precious guide on your quest for a vision. Many blessings to you on your journey!

Training #39
Primal Connection—The Earth-Body Rite of Passage

To begin, I want to make it perfectly clear that even though the physical aspects of the rite of passage I am about to describe—being submerged in the ground overnight—may seem scary or even dangerous to some people, when performed correctly it is absolutely safe. I have personally passed through this rite at least a dozen times, and since 1999 I have led this rite for individuals and groups well over fifty times. Portions of this rite (except highly personal moments) were filmed and aired in 2008 by the History Channel in a ninety-minute special called *Primal Fear*.

The key aspects of this rite of passage are purification, heightened awareness, and visionary experiences fostered through spending one whole night embraced by the earth in a gravelike hole that is dug by hand into the living soil. The experience of intentionally digging your own tomb and being buried in the ground overnight has been described by many who have passed through this rite as a combination of a vision quest and a full-body meditation; it feels like a return to the womb of your true mother to reclaim that mystical union where all of your hurts are purged and absorbed into the immense physical body and energy of the earth. You are then rebirthed into the light of the world to walk a life path infused with the unconditional love and spiritual guidance of Mother Earth.

When performed with proper preparation and in the appropriate manner, the structure of this rite of passage provides an extremely safe and potent opportunity to touch the primal awareness of your entire human organism to such a level that it can truly change your life. Even if you were to simply prepare for the rite, dig and enter your tomb, and then fall asleep for the whole night, you will still be changed. There is no way that one can pass through this rite without being transformed to some degree. However, if you genuinely enter the experience and follow the time-tested suggestions for distilling the most from the rite, the transformational aspects and opportunities for growth and knowledge are limitless.

The earth-body rite of passage is paradoxically very straightforward and extremely complex. The physical side of the ritual is quite simple, and once you learn and understand the logistics you can quickly become comfortable and at ease with the physical aspects of what you are doing and how to do it properly and safely. However, on the mental, psychic, and spiritual levels, the range and complexity of possible experiences prohibits one from knowing or predicting what will actually occur in those realms. The best that one can do for another person performing this rite is to provide a time-tested structure for the ritual along with complete and unconditional support. Of course, there is no substitute for experience in this type of ritual, and having someone to guide the rite who has passed through it multiple times is immensely helpful, although not absolutely necessary. My first time I did it with just a close friend to tend the fire all night.

Here I will describe the rite so that you, together with a friend or small group, can perform the rite in a safe and effective way. If doing this with a group of people, each person digs his or her own tomb, and at least one person remains available to provide external support while the other group members are in their tombs. An extended explanation with dozens of comments from participants can be found in my book *Ecoshamanism: Sacred Practices of Unity, Power and Earth Healing.* However, at the time I wrote that book (2003–2004) I was not yet engaged in formal autogenic training. The evolution of the rite with the addition of AT gives it even more transformative power, and this new version is the one I'm going to share with you here. So let's get started.

The place where you will carry out the rite is extremely important because it is not just the physical location of the rite but also the co-creator of your experience. Optimally, it should be a place that is far enough from civilization that there are no noises from human activity reaching the place and where other people are not going to wander into during the rite. When choosing the site keep in mind that you will be digging into the ground at least two feet deep, so choose a location that has some type of topsoil or sand, not bare rock. You should test the site beforehand by digging a few pilot holes or even a full tomb to make sure the area will be suitable. Be sure to check the area thoroughly to avoid anthills, gopher or other animal holes, snake nests, etc. Also, never perform this rite in an area near a cemetery or archeological site.

Once the site is chosen you must decide exactly where the tomb will be located and positioned, and where the fire will be. If only one tomb is being dug I suggest that the tomb face east, toward the rising sun. If there are multiple tombs being dug as with a group of people, I suggest you place the tombs in a circle around the central fire so the positioning of the tombs resembles the rays of the sun coming out from the fire. In both cases the tomb(s) are approximately five paces from the fire, and while lying in the tomb the body of the initiate is positioned with the head in the part of the tomb closest to the fire. The tomb is rectangular in shape and slightly longer and wider than the person going into it. To set the dimensions of the tomb, simply lie on your back and have someone mark out the outline of the tomb on the surface of the ground using a stick, pick, or shovel. Mark out an area approximately four inches larger than your body all the way around.

Now use whatever hand tools are necessary to dig the tomb(s). I prefer a pick adze and sturdy shovel. While digging, place the soil at the feet side of the tomb, and not between the tomb and the fire. To measure the correct depth of the tomb lie down inside the tomb while lying on your side. Have a friend place a board on the ground and over your shoulder that is facing up. The board should be very close to your shoulder but not touching it. This way you can either lie comfortably on your back during the night or on your side. Be sure to carefully check your tomb for size by actually lying in it. There should be two to four inches extra space all around your body but NOT more or you will lose some of the energetic qualities of the soil encapsulating you.

Once the digging is complete, construct the roof by placing branches or wood planks across the top of the tomb from side to side (NOT front to back). Once the supports for the roof are in place, the easiest way to cover the roof so that when earth is placed on top it doesn't sift through into the tomb is to place a piece of natural cloth (hemp fabric or cotton bedsheets work fine) over the top of the tomb's roof, making sure it is large enough to extend at least six inches over the tomb on all sides. For this stage you can also use natural materials such as leaves, pine needles, field grass, etc., but keep in mind that the last step in constructing the tomb is to completely cover the roof of the tomb with soil, so the roof will have to be able to hold the weight of the soil and also keep it from sifting into the tomb on top of you.

To complete the roof, shovel earth onto it so as to cover the whole tomb with at least 3 inches of earth EXCEPT for an opening just large enough for you to get into at the head of the tomb where you will enter. This section will be covered with earth (except for an opening for air approximately four inches by four inches) by the fire keeper after you are inside the tomb.

Preparation

It is a good idea to prepare your body for the experience by treating it well in the days prior to the burial. Avoid overeating and intoxication. Try to walk and breath intentionally and in a way that improves clarity of thought and action. If you have experience with fasting, this is an appropriate supplement to the burial, but keep in mind that whether you have fasted before or not, you will need sufficient energy for the hard physical work of preparing your tomb. It's a good idea to reduce your water intake in the hours before the burial to reduce the chance of having to urinate. During almost two decades that I have facilitated and participated in this rite of passage no one has ever needed to come out of his tomb during the night for any reason.

In the days prior to the rite you will also have to prepare the material items you will need. These include:

- Materials for taking notes
- Clothes and shoes appropriate for the season and for working outdoors (digging)
- Extra changes of clothes and shoes
- Raingear (in case of wet weather)
- Sunscreen
- Hat for sun protection
- Bottle of water
- Work gloves
- Flashlight with new batteries
- A shovel for digging
- Branches or planks, and cloth for the roof of the tomb
- A pick, adze, or combination pick adze (my favorite)
- Materials for starting a fire and enough wood to keep it burning all night
- Sleeping mat or camping pad or extra blanket to lie on during the night
- Sleeping bag or blanket for warmth
- Pillow if you want one
- Offerings and personal items (such as photos or sacred objects) to take into the tomb

Keep in mind that from the very first moment you decide to enter this rite of passage the sacred ritual has commenced. Everything you do from this moment until you come out of your tomb will affect your experience, so proceed with common sense, intention, and honesty. Many questions and fears are likely to be rolling around in your head. That's good. They are all part of the rite. The more unsure you are about the perceived risks, the greater the possibility for growth and the more lasting the effects of the experience will be. Center your attention on steadily using your fears and insecurities to focus on your preparation.

The Dig

The physical aspects of this rite of passage are just as important as the other levels. If we were to hire a machine to come and dig the tombs we would lose an incalculable amount of insights and lessons that come as a result of digging our own grave. On many levels the digging of the tomb becomes a mirror reflecting the realities of birth, life, death, and rebirth. Many times the insights gleaned while digging the tomb are the most powerful of the whole experience.

The Fire

The transition from day to night marks a corresponding transition in the focus of the activities in this rite of passage. During the day we physically prepare both the tombs as well as our physical body by taking a little food, water, and if available a cleansing bath or shower and change of clothes after the tombs are prepared. When darkness begins to fall we begin to switch from the physically inspired processes to the more numinous levels of awareness as we prepare mentally, emotionally, energetically, and spiritually to enter the womb of the earth during the night. Assisting us in this is the energy, light, heat, and music of the sacred fire. The fire watches over us throughout the night just as the sun did during the day. Thus the fire becomes our night sun.

In this rite, as in most primal activities, the fire plays a significant role in the proceedings. In chapter 13, training #37 is an exercise in how to work in a primal way with fire; I suggest you refer to this training and use the primal techniques with fire included there before entering the tomb for the night. There needs to be at least one person who can stay up all night with the fire while the initiate(s) is in the ground. This fire keeper insures that a small fire is kept alive all night, and that the person(s) in the ground is okay. The fire keeper should not speak to the initiate(s) during the night. The support person can periodically use a drum for a few minutes at a time throughout the night. The beat of the drum should not be any sort of "music." A slow, steady beat resembling a heartbeat is best.

On Dying and Being Reborn

In this rite of passage we intentionally pursue circumstances that bring out from within us the transformational power that is fostered through metaphorically dying and being reborn. But unlike other spiritual forms of this process wherein the metaphor is drawn up through words or commitments of being born again, in this rite we actually dig a grave and submerge ourselves in it, thereby facing our mortality with our entire primal human organism. This is about as close as you can get to the awareness of death without placing yourself in mortal danger or having a physical near-death experience. Also, in this ritual context you are totally submerged inside an organic process and provided with the support and encouragement to take the opportunity to make positive use of the experience in a way that improves the quality of your life and happiness. In his book *The Unfolding Self*, psychologist Ralph Metzner, an expert on transformative experience, gets right to the point with respect to the implications of the death-rebirth initiation:

> Whereas in some Christian fundamentalist circles it is customary for people who have made a commitment to Christ to refer to themselves as "twice born," the original meaning of that concept goes much deeper than simply a profession of renewed faith, however sincere. It refers, actually, to the second part of a death-rebirth transformational process. The rebirth experience, to be authentic, must of necessity be preceded by an experience of metaphorically dying. This first, dying phase is inevitably anxiety provoking and problematical for most people. . . . In the mystery religions of ancient times and in

many traditional cultures, "death-rebirth" was and is the name of an initiatory experience. Associated with it are the ritual practices such as entombment, profound isolation, or painful ordeal through which the initiate must pass. Afterward, the initiate customarily adopts a new name, perhaps a new garment, and sometimes a new role in society, all of which express the newly reborn being.[1]

The Tomb

The initiate climbs into the tomb and the material world is left behind. A threshold to the shamanic world of nature and spirit is crossed. The immediate and familiar supports of family, friends, colleagues, pets, accomplishments, failures, and all the trappings and freedoms of everyday life are severed. As the initiate lies down in the tomb, the tomb becomes a sacred chamber consecrated by the concrete action of the initiate to know both self and world in new and improved ways. Lying in the tomb with the entrance having been covered by the fire keeper, the flesh of the initiate is formally offered to the body of the earth. In these moments, as the last shovels-full of soil are being thrown on top of the tomb, the exchange between the initiate and the earth begins. Flesh begins to become soil, and soil begins to become flesh. All begins to come together as one.

The preparations over, now it is just you, the earth, and the journey you are about to take inside and out. The fire keeper has opened a fist-size hole in the corner of the roof of your earthly cocoon. You are not trapped, and you will not die this night. This airhole insures that fresh life-giving air surrounds you and is inside of you. The love of the earth is embracing you. The energy of the fire is protecting you. The rest of your life is waiting for you. The fire keeper puts his hand through the airhole and into the tomb. You take his hand in yours, the feelings of life and love, companionship, and kinship flow between you. And then the hand is gone. The journey begins . . .

And so the journey, so unique and personal to each initiate, begins as the settling-in process continues and the fears, anxieties, hopes, and dreams begin to increase and dissipate as this passage unfolds. The experiences in the earth-body are as unique as the individuals, the lessons as profound as the mysteries of life. At this stage of the ritual it is common to pass through a period of questioning or even rage or feelings of depression. In many cases but certainly not all this phase is actually very conducive to later in the night experiencing profound insights or visions. This period of doubt is another threshold to cross over once one is actually inside the tomb, and once it is crossed a new hallway opens up in front of you with many more rooms to explore.

Once one passes through these initial phases of the ritual, sleep sometimes comes as the person becomes more comfortable with the surroundings and with him- or herself. From this point the initiate passes through different levels, between fully awake and fully asleep. In my experience this is usually the most productive way to spend the night during this ritual because you get to experience many different levels and states of consciousness, which is also one reason for periods of drumming throughout the night, as the sound of the beating drum facilitates shifts in consciousness. Although the experience of sleeping throughout the night in the tomb has its own benefits, shifting between being awake and asleep, and all the levels in between, has proven to be the most useful format for first-time initiates.

Once you have settled in I suggest that you perform a full session of standard AT formulas to fully connect with your physical body. After doing that, throughout the night use any other formulas from the many you have learned—affirmation formulas, healing formulas, visualization formulas, and tunnel formulas. If you have followed the AT process with me during the course of this book you have the perfect chance in this rite to use your knowledge and experience with AT in a unique and transformative setting.

As we did in the advanced AT training, this rite provides you with an extremely novel and powerful situation for asking questions and passively receiving answers. It's perfectly fine to use your flashlight intermittently and review your questions from your notebook, or look at any photos you brought with you. This is no time to be shy with yourself.

Along with performing the standard and advanced AT formulas, the question-and-answer dialog while submerged in the earth has been found to be very effective, especially for those who are passing through a difficult time in life. These questions are of the most personal nature, and experience has shown that the more specific the question the more specific the answer. Generally phrased questions usually receive general or vague responses.

Throughout my years of listening to initiates describe the question-and-answer process that goes on inside the tomb, one of the striking parallels is between the outcome of the dialog and the transformational metaphor of passing from fragmentation to wholeness. This is a recurrent theme in primal rites of passage as well as ancient mystical traditions and stems from the idea that fragmented parts of our psyche can be joined together and made whole again, thereby moving a person from a disjointed or confused state of being into a more harmonious and centered perspective. This is a particularly valuable experience, especially for our lives in the modern, fast-paced world where we sometimes feel split and scattered and not sure if we are coming or going. Our modern lives so frequently ask that we wear many different hats all at the same time, and often these separate roles are at odds with one another and we end up feeling torn and pulled and stretched to the breaking point.

There is an unlimited number of experiences that can occur when in the ground for a night. It is always amazing to me how being isolated and enclosed so often leads to out-of-body or even flying experiences. During the core segments of this ritual it is quite common to feel like you're out of your body, looking down on your tomb or the fire. Sometimes this leads to a feeling or perception of transition between one level of consciousness and another. Initiates also often describe moving through or down a tunnel that leads to a transition that fosters feelings of serenity, peace, unity, love, or even ecstasy. Some people even describe seeing or visiting with dead relatives or friends. Once in a half-sleep, half-awake state in the tomb I had a significant vision and conversation with my father, who had passed when I was fifteen. During that conversation I was fourteen and he was still alive and healthy. Other people report receiving complex yet meaningful visions about life and our connection to the living earth.

Feelings or visions of disintegrating into the soil are also fairly common, as is the life review. This phenomenon is in many ways similar to a near-death experience, in which during the course of only a few seconds their lives flash before them like a movie run at superhigh speed. This type of life review spurred by a near-death experience often results in an awakening within the person that marks a major turning point in life, with subsequent changes in lifestyle and a deepening of relationships at a personal level.

Having personally passed through four separate near-death experiences (two as a result of automobile accidents, one from a rock-climbing incident, and one at the hands of the Huichol peyote), and also having had such experiences while buried in the earth, I can say at least for me that there are similarities between the two experiences but also some significant differences. The near-death experience life review is superfast, even though while you are living it it may seem much longer. Although each of my four life-review experiences brought on by near-death experiences were unique in feeling, in many ways they all felt like a sort of purging of my conscious life experiences before my consciousness could move to another realm or be obliterated. In each case the awareness that the end of what I call "me" was about to happen was undeniably real, and the resulting effects (as of course I didn't die) were powerful to the point that in each case I came from the experience a changed person with renewed motivations and inspiration.

In contrast, initiates who have a life-review experience in the tomb usually compare it more to what it would be like in the last few days or hours of a terminally ill person. In this case the person approaches death gradually and has the chance (if she takes it) to review her life more slowly, to make amends with people, resolve inner conflicts, etc. In fact, sometimes afterward initiates complain that during a life-review experience they got "stuck" when reviewing a life situation they never fully dealt with, sometimes in a very uncomfortable spot. This is something I've never heard of during the life-review in a near-death experience. Also, it is often reported during the life-review in this rite that life experiences that were apparently forgotten by the initiate were suddenly resurrected, and in most cases the forgotten moments were very poignant to the future growth of the person.

Another significant aspect to the earth-body rite is that the unique qualities of the soil and being buried in the earth come together to form an experience that is so grounded it directly promotes the gathering up and pulling together of the splintered and fragmented pieces of our psyche and soul. This process is often described as a "reremembering" of who you really are. Healing from fragmentation also comes in another manner as we see that the splinters of our life are not just pieces formed from attempting too many activities at once (so-called multitasking), it also results from intentionally or unintentionally hiding those parts of ourselves we can't or don't want to face. Without going into a long discussion about Jungian shadow philosophy, suffice it to say that reconciling with the shadow aspects of one's psyche is in many ways facilitated by the earth-body rite of passage. This happens in myriad ways, but one common component seems to be that being in the tomb for an extended period of time places everything in perspective. While in the ground everything comes together and becomes equal. Everything is equally relevant and irrelevant. There is no one on whom I can project my feelings, and no one there for me to mirror. My mirror is the earth, and my reflection is the universe.

In terms of moving from fragmentation to wholeness, or reconciling with our hidden or shadow sides, the earth-body rite almost always has a positive influence as these themes are integrated into the initiates' lives after they leave their tombs. The underlying physical structure of the rite simply perpetuates wholeness and grounding. In some way the earthy cocoon of the grave compresses our energetic field so that even if we don't have visions or receive answers we still come out feeling different—more confident, at ease, peaceful. Some describe it as being engulfed in the loving embrace of the earth. Others feel it as overcoming their greatest fears or pulling through a great challenge. Here is a short passage written by Susan after the rite:

> My time in the womb of the earth was an experience I will never forget, and it has been a gift to me every day since I did it. Looking back, I have never felt so peaceful as that night wrapped in the arms of my true mother. I felt safe, and strangely comfortable. My tomb/womb was a miraculous gift from the Goddess. It is permanently etched in my mind. Every rock (even the ones sticking in my back that I hated then but love now), every root, every hue of clay, soil, and mud, every smell and sound I will never forget. My lesson was that I can be loved, that I deserve to be loved, and that I want to be loved. Mother Earth gave me an awesome gift—she woke me up silently and without me even knowing . . .

Emergence

It may sound hard to believe but when the sun rises and the time has finally come to get out of the tomb many people don't want to leave just yet. After spending the whole night in their cocoon it has become part of them, or they of it. With the morning light of a new day streaming in through the air hole the tomb doesn't seem quite so menacing or intense. When leading a group through this rite of passage I always try to feel how the group is doing in the moments right before emergence and weigh that against the experiences of the night. Does it feel like one member of the group needs or wants to come out first, or right away? Or does it feel like they want or need to stay in the tomb a little while longer? Normally it is clear how long to wait. When the time comes I go to the first tomb and gently tell the initiate that it's time to emerge. I give brief instructions as to how I will get them out, tell them to cover their eyes, and as a last instruction I suggest that when the passage is made for them to come out, and they are ready, to crawl out of the tomb, stand up with their arms and fingers outstretched to the sky, and pronounce, "HERE I AM, FOR THE FIRST TIME!" or something similar.

Janet wrote this in her notebook just before being taken out of the tomb:

The answers to my questions, my visions, hopes, and dreams, came to me during the night in the form of many songs. My latest song came in the predawn light as the little birds began to sing in the trees near to the grave site, and I heard a flock of geese fly overhead. Even though I had a few rough moments during the night and some of my songs were accompanied by great pain and remorse, now that the time draws near to come out I feel like I could stay in here a long time more. Especially if I had a yogurt and some fresh water!

Now I can actually hear the others being taken out of the tombs. Some of them are greeting the sun and singing. I don't feel like coming out. It's so nice and cozy in here. Now that the rite is over I wish I could just stay in here and sleep for a few hours. Or is it that I don't want to face the world just yet? Being with people has never been very easy for me. I need another song, a song of rebirth, of a new life. James just came and I asked him if I can stay a few more minutes. I'm not ready yet . . .

Although in some cases such as the above experience of Janet I allow an initiate some extra time in the tomb, for first-time initiates it is extremely important that they rebirth, emerge from the womb, and cut the umbilical cord as part of the ritual and in the company of both the living beings of the land and their human companions. Too many adults of our culture are adolescents in adult bodies. This ritual marks a significant transformation for those people, and for the others it is important to simply put the experiences of the tomb in perspective and walk out into the world to begin reintegration.

At this point in the ritual many possibilities emerge. In the best-case scenario we would have at least the whole day to fill in the tombs, perform a rite that incorporates submerging in the water of a stream or lake, sharing a light meal, and discussing the trials and tribulations of integrating the experiences of the burial into our daily lives. At the very least we restore the area as closely as we can to how we found it and have a brief discussion before departing. In any case, the first hour or two after you emerge from the tomb will be very special. Words appear in the air again, hugs are received and given, laughter and smiles are shared, and the eyes of your companion(s) will reflect your journey. You are back in the world of people, and now the most difficult part of the ritual has begun: taking your experience with you and not forgetting.

Integration

While integrating back into society you must not let your visions disperse or be rendered useless by letting the world of others suck them dry. While at first it is normal to feel happy about emerging and being with people again, it is important to remember that you emerge from the tomb in a highly receptive and vulnerable energetic state. You are like a child again in the sense of being very impressionable and innocent. The ritual time has cleansed away a large portion of your normal defenses and left your true primal being to shine out ever more brightly. Now the trick is to remain shining.

Upon your return home you will probably feel glad but also alienated. You had left home to go find something and now that you are back you are not the same. While you and your home were once one and the same, now you are different, and so you begin walking in two different worlds. The first world is the sacred time of the rite of passage that you just passed through, your magic time spent with the living soil and fire, sun and wind, with your companions and with your spirit. But the second world of "civilized" people and schedules is calling you back and you must go. That is the way it is—you go to the rite of passage to submerge in the first world and be born anew into the second. Now your job begins as you walk back into the second world and try to balance it with the first. Along the way it will help you to reconnect with the experiences of the rite of passage by periodically going to a quiet place in nature and reflecting on the process as you place your hands in the soil. In this way you can keep the experience close to your heart and also give yourself an opportunity to remember, relive, or integrate any experiences of the rite that may have remained obscure for any reason. Another way to do this is to reconnect with the fire that was present that whole night, even if with only a candle.

Once your visions have been internalized, you walk the world carrying them with you, but now it is up to you to make them manifest in the world. This requires action. It is very rare when a rite of passage provides all the answers or visions that you are seeking; the rite is an ongoing process, and it helps you to see what you couldn't before and spurs you onward. Sometimes you will stumble, but it is in those moments when the energy of the rite is there for you. The rite has shown you your true potential, and nothing can stop you from emerging. I received this note from Anne a few months after she underwent the rite:

> Re-entry into my life has been difficult. I had a long drive home, which helped. I kept yelling out the car window "Here I am for the first time!" The colors of the trees, bright reds, yellows, rusts, felt like big hands holding me, and I had tears in my eyes thinking about how loving and supportive Mother Earth is to us. As I drove into town, the first thing I saw was a man throwing his cigarette butt out his car window. I was furious, honked and yelled at him not to do that. I felt very protective of the Earth Mother and was thrown back into my life right away. I kept thinking about wanting to be back inside the earth.
>
> I've made considerable effort to continue the exercise of the five gates with the fire, and I've dealt directly with my mom and dad and my ex to realize the dream visions of my tomb. I've been disappointed but also made good progress in some other things in my life. Months later the experience is still very much a part of me, it is embedded in my psyche, and I continue to reflect on the entire experience. It is nothing less than amazing and I can't wait to do it again. I can't say that all of my prayers and questions have been answered, however, I do know that participating in the rite has helped me discover what I may not have been able to otherwise. And that is a great gift . . . THANK YOU!

15

PRIMAL MIND OF
THE COSMIC CLOWNS

I first met Highwater, a revered holy man of the Arapahoe tribe, when I was in my late teens. I was hitchhiking to my job at a ski resort in Colorado, and he picked me up on a nearly deserted back road near where I was living. I had no idea who he was, and in that moment I really didn't care. It was freezing, and I was just thankful for the ride. But our connection was immediate. He showed me kindness and respect and gave me some warm coffee from his thermos.

Highwater was an extraordinary man. Through the years he shared with me many ancient and sacred items of his people that few whites had ever seen. Every time he picked me up hitchhiking it was like a sacred meeting, and he would share some bit of wisdom that I would use during the course of my day. I was delighted when many years later he was to come to my home so that I could return some of the favors he had given to me in the past. I had arranged for him to do some talks and maybe healing sessions in and around Sedona, where I lived at the time. He was happy to make some money for his grandmother who was ill; even though she didn't want the money it would help buy food and other things for her ceremony when she died. Anyway, Highwater was coming from Colorado, and I knew that with Highwater it was not going to be a picnic. Granted, he was quick to laugh and joke around, but his methods of teaching were equally powerful. I knew in my gut that something big would happen when he visited.

The night he arrived it was very late, and we shared a couple of sips of whisky on my couch in front of the fire of my woodstove. Then he unrolled his blanket, curled up on the couch, and said goodnight. But just as I turned away he sat up and with an intense look said, "Sweet dreams." I didn't think much of that comment and went to bed and quickly fell asleep. That night I had lucid dreams of thunder and lightning and a giant horse that ran right at me and struck me down. Then it turned and ran back and trampled me to death. I awakened from this dream in the middle of the night and walked out to the kitchen to get some water. I was so focused on drinking water I didn't notice Highwater as I walked through the living room to get my water. But after I chugged two glasses down and turned to go back to bed, I saw Highwater sitting up on the couch, staring into the fire.

"Come here and sit, boy," he said in a faraway voice.

I sat next to this holy man, and he asked me what I had just dreamed. I told him what I had seen, and he let out a big sigh. He put his face in his hands and bent over as if feeling terribly sad. But for some reason I felt like he was simply pretending to be sad, and that he was actually grinning inside.

"You have dreamt of the opposite ones. This is powerful medicine that cannot be ignored. It is one of the most difficult tests in the life of a medicine man. Now you have to live the life of a contrary. Everything you do must be the opposite of everything you know. This seems silly to "civilized" people, but it is one of the most sacred acts to us Apache. The Hopi also do it in their kachina dances, where the clown, the opposite, makes fun of everything. But in his fun-making he is one of the most sacred dancers. To our relatives, the Dakota, when someone has a dream like yours they become *heyoka,* a thunder being that completely reverses typical behavior, for that is how one sees the second world, the world that others are blind to. In our Apache tradition outsiders see the heyoka as a clown, a mere joke, but the sacred fool embodies the

paradox of life and to us is seen as sacred. There is nothing more difficult than to be your opposite, and any man who can do it will eventually *see* the world with new eyes and embrace the cosmic paradox. This
is what you will begin to do right now. You want to sit here by the fire
with me, but now you need to get naked and sit outside in the dark and
cold. Take off all your clothes and GO NOW!"

I was totally bewildered by Highwater's words. I didn't want to go
out into the cold, dark night, especially naked. But I did it anyway. I
stripped and lay on the couch on my front porch. There was already a
blanket there, so I was relieved for that, and I brought my best friend,
Sophie, my female German shepherd, out with me, and we both curled
up. Not five minutes later Highwater came out onto the porch, took my
blanket, and took Sophie inside with him.

"You are heyoka now," he said sternly. "You get no warmth, no comfort from your dog, and NO sleep." He handed me a piece of manzanita
wood, also known as ironwood because it is so hard, and a small pocket
knife. "Whittle on this wood until the sun comes up, and if I catch you
sleeping I swear to god I will put you over my knee and spank you!"

I had no doubt in my mind that Highwater would do exactly what
he had promised, so I whittled that branch to nothing while shivering
so hard in the cold that when the dawn came I was never so happy
in my life. When he finally came out the front door onto the porch,
Highwater, to my great relief, had a kind look on his face and was carrying my coffee mug. I couldn't wait to put my cold hands on it and drink
the warm brew. But instead of handing me a nice hot cup of coffee he
threw an ice-cold cup of water in my face!

"Hahahahah! You are heyoka now, you little pissant! Now get in
your truck and wait for me; we're going for a ride."

"But I have no clothes on!"

"That's right . . . And that's why it's going to be so incredibly fun!"

I was livid. But I walked to my truck naked, started it, and turned
the heater on full blast as I sat in the driver's seat barely able to keep my
eyes open. Highwater entered the truck soon after, slapped me hard in

the face, as he could see I was falling asleep, and immediately turned off the truck heater and rolled down all the windows. He was dressed in my warmest goose-down coat that he must have gotten from my closet, warm boots, and even gloves and a hat. Of course I was still completely naked. He then had me drive into town to buy gas. When we arrived at the station he said he would go inside and pay so I wouldn't get arrested, but that I was to pump the gas. Incredibly, and I can't say how, the few other people at the gas station never even noticed me. Then Highwater took me to a popular tourist hiking trail at the base of Cathedral Rock, and I walked the whole trail, about two hours, passing more than a few people, and not one person said anything about my nakedness.

When we got home, Highwater told me to get dressed in my best suit and tie (I only owned one, for weddings and funerals). And later that night we went to a local bookstore that friends of mine owned. This was where Highwater was to give a talk, and the place was packed. I knew more than half the people there, and I was the brunt of more than a few jokes and funny looks. Of course Highwater knew no one would be wearing a suit except me and how out of place I would look in a suit and tie at a New Age bookstore, and me being the local hiking guide at that! The ego is a tricky animal, and my dream was interpreted by him as meaning that I needed to be broken down, to become more humble, to not be ashamed of being naked or looking like the fool.

Later when we got home that night—and by the way he did not let me talk on the drive home because he knew that's exactly what I wanted to do—he made me sleep in my suit, and in the morning he shook me awake. For the next week he made me do and say everything the opposite. I could sleep in the day but not at night. When he asked me a question I had to say no when I wanted to say yes. I had to shit outside where there was an ant hole so they would crawl on me while I did my business. Cold showers. No phone calls. No computer. No visitors. Daily walks through town walking backward (but at least not naked anymore). Then he took me up to the Yavapai reservation and put this mask on my face that looked like a seagull on acid, and he paraded me around the reservation while telling me to flap my arms like a bird. I could see out of the small eyeholes of this ridiculous mask, so I could see and hear all the people laughing at me. But truth be told, I didn't care anymore. The ridicule was sacred. These people knew what Highwater was doing to me. They laughed anyway because it was still damn funny to see this white guy in a silly bird mask dancing around flapping his wings with an old holy man kicking him in the butt the whole time.

After strolling me around the whole village, Highwater instructed the children who were following us to go get buckets of water. They created a giant mudhole in the middle of the village; then they all surrounded me, and I had flashbacks of being in a large mosh pit at a rock concert. To my dismay, the biggest warriors of the tribe came along and began throwing me into the mud. Every time I would stagger up they threw me in again until I was a totally muddy mess. Then, to my utter surprise, most of the young warriors stripped off all their clothes, the children stripped me of mine, and for the next half hour or so we had a crazy mud brawl naked in the mud. All ego was left behind. Naked men playing in the mud tackling one another, throwing mud at one another, with no maliciousness, just pure, unadulterated fun of the kind rarely experienced by "civilized" people.

Afterward, Highwater took a hose and hosed us all clean. After we were dressed, the men both young and old all gave me hugs and said, "You are now heyoka, a cosmic clown without inhibitions, just like us. Next time someone comes to be heyoka you are welcome to come and dance the mud bath with us."*

The sacred fool is a very important and powerful figure in almost every primal culture in North America and in many others I have visited throughout the globe. Sometimes during ceremonies or certain times of year there will be more than one sacred clown ritualizing and satirizing

---

*This is an abridged version of the story but makes the point. For the whole story and twenty-five more stories of my experiences with shamans and primal elders, see my book *Lightning in My Blood*.

human behavior. The cosmic clowns possess extraordinary power and privilege. They have full license to express outlandish, outrageous behavior, and no one, not even the chiefs and holy men and women, can escape them. In fact, the leaders of the tribe are the ones the clowns usually pick on the most! But unlike most of our modern ego-inflated leaders, these primal elders know the importance of poking fun and fooling around. They are usually the ones laughing the hardest at themselves.

I have also seen in certain moments the whole community of people openly participate as temporary clowns. In this way the whole world is shaken to its core. I have found this again and again among primal people; they live inside this amazing reality where every action has meaning and everything is sacred, while at the same time nothing, absolutely nothing, is above jest, ridicule, absurdity, and humor.

In the spirit of the cosmic clown I'm going to leave you with this final primal training. Although to outsiders the primal clowns appear many times to be engaged in totally inappropriate behavior,* their core mission is simply to illuminate that which may be obscure or hidden, whether intentionally or not. This has been called "inverting the world" by ethnologist Holger Kalweit, in his studies of primal shamans:

> The primal healer . . . lives in a world that lies at a remove from our own and that appears to us as twisted or mad. [He] is a fool who turns everything upside down, but he is a holy fool. He is holy because he has been healed, because he has gone beyond illness and deception. In light of this, we may ask which world is the inverted one—theirs or ours?[1]

We can see the essence of the cosmic clown in modern times in the lifestyle of voluntary simplicity of author, educator, and activist

---

*I must note here that I have never seen anyone physically hurt by the sacred clowns, such as lying or stealing or rape or murder; it's more a sense of tomfoolery. Those appointed to be clowns are mature members of the community and know their role is not to harm but to illuminate.

Duane Elgin;[2] in the classic and noble truths of Buddhist scholar Rick Fields and colleagues;[3] and in the many modern Thoreaus, Emersons, Aldo Leopolds, and John Muirs of our times, and of course the cross-cultural traditional medicine and practices of Clarissa Pinkola Estés and modern ecofeminists. I could go on and on about the contributions so many forward-thinking people are currently making. I feel I am doing them an injustice by not naming them, but there's simply no room here. In any case, you know who you are, and because in some respect I know you I also know most of you would prefer to be unnamed.

Now, on to the final training of this book:

Training #40
Inverting the World

All of the training practices in this book directly or indirectly relate to this theme of the cosmic clown, whose specialty is to invert the world and expand awareness and perception, allowing us to do things we have probably never been told to do. In our culture we are normally not taught about the possibilities and health benefits of self-regulating our bodies, passive and concentrated visualization, using affirmations to change harmful behaviors or accomplish goals, meditating with our subtle body's energy tunnels, reawaking our senses, or embracing the world of nature with our primal mind. None of these activities go with the flow of the predictable Western mind.

I choose the word *predictable* simply because we have been coerced into thinking conformity is the only reality. Even in just my own lifetime I have seen this transformation. I can scarcely imagine what someone one hundred years old has seen. The time of the town square as a center of activity is all but gone, replaced by chain stores and shopping malls. I recently traveled by car from California to the East Coast. It's amazing how simple it is now to know when you've reached the next town: as soon as you see the local Walmart and the area's popular fast-food chain, you know you have arrived.

This homogenizing of our culture has been described by historian Theodore Roszak* as "single vision." This relatively new single vision, according to Roszak, is an artificial result of narrowed possibilities. It is objective in the sense that this single vision is necessary in order to allow the exploitation of the planet, and one another, as objects. Older, more primal cultures live in a world of subjectivity. The subjective view of reality ties the human community together and the human communities to nature. When we get to a place of subjectivity we can let go of the data, standards, and statistics, and simply realize *This is how it feels to be me.* This awareness is direct, subjective, and unfiltered by beliefs or outside interpretations.

In this sense, all the trainings in this book are subjective in nature and "multi-visional." So I invite you to carry on with the untypical practices. These practices (trainings) can be called *inversion practices, counter-practices,* or *cosmic-clown training.* For those of you familiar with the books of Carlos Castaneda, they would be termed *not-doings.* In any case, having a name for something doesn't mean we know it. Our cosmic-clown training of inverting the world is basically the intentional doing of something in a way other than our habitual way. Some of these are simple and easy, but they still place us in a subjective experience of perceiving in new ways. They shift our personal perspective and in some cases can powerfully illuminate our subtle body and be felt in our energy tunnels (or chakras). As an added bonus, some of them can turn out to be quite fun! Here are some examples. As always, I suggest you try the following examples and then take this experience to another level by creating your own.

"Our belief at the beginning of a doubtful undertaking," says the great American psychologist William James in *The Varieties of Religious Experience,* "is the one thing that ensures the successful outcome of the venture."

---

*Roszak (1933–2011) was a well-known author on topics of counterculture, information systems, and ecopsychology. He was professor emeritus of history at California State University.

- Create something beautiful and then give it away to someone you don't know and will probably never see again. While you are giving it you may feel regret, but you will learn that you need not possess something to own it.
- With the help of a friend for safety, blindfold yourself for twenty-four hours while still performing many functions of your everyday life.
- Walk backward for a half hour each day for a week.
- Take a tape recorder with you and record yourself during various conversations and situations. Is that really you?
- Tell a total stranger a secret that you've never told anyone before.
- Tell yourself lies in front of a mirror. Tell yourself how great you are, how good-looking, how intelligent, smart, funny, successful . . . After a while the lies and the truths are all the same. Do it now.
- Read out loud all the ingredients of the packaged food you eat each time before you eat it.
- Put the specialness back into simple items: for a week only use one plate, glass, fork, pair of shoes, socks, or underwear.
- Set an extra place at dinner for three nights (or more). Who would you invite to sit there? Pick anyone from history or your current life. Why did you pick these people? Can you visualize them sitting there eating? What do you talk about?
- Say "thank you" to everything. If you stub your toe say thank you to the kid's toy that caused you pain. Before you start to eat say thank you to your fork. When you drop something say thank you before you pick it up.
- We've all seen the "adopt a highway" signs. What about adopting something really important, like a stream or an old-growth forest?
- Revolt against helium party balloons; they always seem to end up where they don't belong.
- Make peaceful rebellion your church. Revolt against your own self-imposed limitations and those put on you by society. If your

rebellion feels uncomfortable, then you're doing it right.

- Don't speak for at least two days. Spend your time listening instead. Write it out if it's really that important. I do this exercise frequently (my partner doesn't mind a bit), and it's amazing to discover how much I really don't need to say.

- If you are a shy nontalker do the opposite. Plan to go someplace where no one knows you and intentionally be outgoing. It doesn't matter what you say; even if you look foolish, who cares? When surrounded by people who have no idea who you are you can be anyone.

- Just like a child who knows the world is still a mystery, ask the question "Why?" to everything and to everyone.

- Try doing something you think you won't like or seems like a complete waste of time. I did this with the herbal body butter, and now I love it.

- Read *The Man Who Planted Trees,* and then see how it feels to be like him.

- Rearrange all the things in your house, or better yet, have a good friend do it for you.

- Write down one good thing you have ever done in your life.

- Write down your deepest, darkest secret.

- Write down your most secret sexual fantasy.

- Draw a picture of a brain (most of us have seen a picture of a brain). Now draw in *your* lobes. These are not scientific lobes, but instead they depict how much time you spend thinking about certain things. If you think about money or your kids a lot then these lobes will be bigger than a lobe for death, which might be small. Draw and label eight to ten such lobes inside your brain.

- Create something cool, and then destroy it. Tibetan monks, Native Americans, and Australian Aborigines do this all the time with intricate sand paintings.

- Dance like a dervish (Sufi whirling), spinning and whirling around with hands above the head in a physically active meditation.

- Use your nondominant hand for the activities you usually use your dominant hand for. Do this at least for a day. I try to do this at least once a month and sometimes just randomly for fun. It has really helped on those occasions where I have injured my dominant hand/arm.
- Dress up and go out as the opposite sex.
- Think about this: if your house was on fire and you could save only one thing, what would it be? Why?
- If you don't already know, and most people don't, find out where you actually live in terms of nature, not the imaginary human-placed boundaries that are made for purely political reasons. A bioregion is an area bounded by natural rather than artificial borders that has characteristic flora and fauna and includes one or more ecosystems. The most general way of placing where you live in nature is by your watershed. What watershed do you live in? Where does your running water come from?
- Try to sell your stuff to telemarketers when they call you.

One of the most powerful ways to educate yourself, to open your mind to alternative ways of experiencing the world and thus to counteract the influence of social conditioning and the mass media is to read backward. By this I mean to read books printed ten years ago, twenty years ago, fifty years ago, a hundred years ago, two hundred years ago, five hundred years ago, a thousand years ago, or two thousand years ago. When you do so you can step outside the presuppositions and ideologies of the present time and develop an informed world perspective. Or as Ralph Waldo Emerson said, "If we encountered a man of rare intelligence we should ask him what books he read." When you read only in the present, no matter how extensively, you are apt to absorb widely shared misconceptions taught and believed today as the truth. When you read backward, though, you will come to understand some of the stereotypes and misconceptions of the present. You will develop a better sense of what is universal and what is relative, what is essential and what is arbitrary.

The following is a sampling of authors whose writings will enable you to rethink the present, so that you can reshape and expand your worldview. Note: This list of authors represents a decidedly Western worldview. It's recommended that once you have grounded yourself in deeply insightful authors from the Western world, you then read works by the great Eastern authors.

- **More than 2,000 years ago:** Plato, Aristotle, Aeschylus, Aristophanes
- **1200s:** Thomas Aquinas, Dante
- **1300s:** Boccaccio, Chaucer
- **1400s:** Erasmus, Francis Bacon
- **1500s:** Machiavelli, Cellini, Cervantès, Montaigne
- **1600s:** John Milton, Pascal, John Dryden, John Locke, Joseph Addison
- **1700s:** Thomas Paine, Thomas Jefferson, Adam Smith, Benjamin Franklin, Alexander Pope, Edmund Burke, Edward Gibbon, Samuel Johnson, Goethe, Rousseau, William Blake
- **1800s:** Jane Austen, Charles Dickens, Emile Zola, Balzac, Dostoyevsky, Sigmund Freud, Karl Marx, Charles Darwin, John Henry Newman, John Stuart Mill, Leo Tolstoy, the Brontës, Frank Norris, Thomas Hardy, Emile Durkheim, Edmond Rostand, Oscar Wilde, William James
- **1900s:** Ambrose Bierce, Gustavus Myers, H. L. Mencken, William Graham Sumner, W. H. Auden, Bertolt Brecht, Joseph Conrad, Max Weber, Aldous Huxley, Franz Kafka, Sinclair Lewis, Henry James, Jean-Paul Sartre, Virginia Woolf, William Appleman Williams, Arnold Toynbee, C. Wright Mills, Albert Camus, Willa Cather, Bertrand Russell, Karl Mannheim, Thomas Mann, Albert Einstein, Simone De Beauvoir, Winston Churchill, William J. Lederer, Vance Packard, Eric Hoffer, Erving Goffman, Philip Agee, John Steinbeck, Ludwig Wittgenstein, William Faulkner, Talcott Parsons, Jean Piaget, Lester Thurow,

Robert Reich, Robert Heilbroner, Noam Chomsky, Ralph Nader, Margaret Mead, Bronislaw Malinowski, Karl Popper, Robert Merton, Peter Berger, Milton Friedman, J. Bronowski

If you don't have access to an extensive library (or even if you do), really old books can be hard to find. An outstanding online resource is Project Gutenberg (www.gutenberg.org), which offers over 46,000 free e-books. Many of the above authors are included in this collection, especially the oldest ones.

WHAT'S NEXT?

Let's take a moment to briefly consider what we've been doing. We certainly traversed a lot of ground. We learned specific autogenic training techniques and formulas to engage our autonomic nervous system, added affirmation and healing formulas, and explored in novel ways a variety of advanced visualization techniques of inner self-discovery and meditation techniques involving our organs, glands, and energetic tunnels. Taking this knowledge with us we embarked on a journey of reawakening our natural senses and walking the path of primal awareness in nature. Finally, we "clowned around" for a while. The combining of autogenic training and primal-mind awareness supplied us with a comprehensive psychophysiological system of personal growth to help propel us forward to optimum health, heightened awareness, and hopefully a renewed sense of happiness.

So what's next? Well, I know I have never read a book of techniques concerning personal growth and completed them all. Maybe you have, and congratulations are thus in order. However, for those of you who are more like me, you might want to try the techniques you skipped. I have found that in many cases the things we avoid are the things we need the most. Also, this book is so crammed full of training practices derived from decades of experience that I always suggest to my workshop participants to keep on practicing. This is not a race with a finish line. To effectively embody all forty of these trainings usually takes folks many years.

It is also my hope that what's next includes your taking my suggestions and personally refining these techniques and creating new ones. I also hope that you will share them with others. Although classic AT is highly personal, we have seen the myriad ways it can be used in combination with PM techniques and connection to nature. Many of these activities are perfect to do with others (especially children). Almost all of the techniques in this book I have done with groups of people. Sure, sometimes a technique will need to be slightly altered, but the core remains.

Before you close this book take a few moments to reflect on your AT-PM experiences. What trainings did you resonate with? Which caused you frustration? Close your eyes, and relive certain experiences that come to you. Think about what trainings you will continue and which ones you will try again to master. I sincerely hope that the information in this book has been valuable to you. Many blessings on *your* journey! —JE

NOTES

1. WHAT IS AUTOGENIC TRAINING?

1. Schultz, *Das Autogene.*
2. Green and Green, *Beyond Biofeedback,* 55.

2. WHAT IS PRIMAL MIND?

1. Cassirer, *Essay on Man.*
2. Highwater, *Primal Mind,* 19.
3. Fredrickson, *Black Image in the White Mind,* 74.
4. Jung, *Psychological Reflections.*

7. AUTOGENIC TRAINING AND MEDICAL/PSYCHOSOMATIC/ PSYCHIATRIC DISORDERS

1. Linden, *Autogenic Training,* 113.

8. VISUALIZATION AND AUTOGENIC TRAINING

1. Schultz and Luthe, *Autogenic Training.*
2. Luthe, *Autogenic Therapy.*

9. APPLYING AUTOGENIC TRAINING TO MEDITATION AND TO THE SUBTLE-ENERGY CENTERS

1. Goodwin, "At the Temple of James Arthur Ray," www.theguardian.com/ world/2011/jul/08/james-arthur-ray-sweat-lodge-arizona.

2. Ibid.

3. Fonseca, "Another Survivor of Sweat Lodge Retreat Speaks," www.azcentral .com/news/articles/2009/10/21/20091021sweatlodgedeaths21-ON.html.

4. Gerber, *Vibrational Medicine,* 83.

5. Motoyama, *Science and the Evolution of Consciousness* cited in ibid., 94–96.

6. Hunt, "Electronic Evidence."

7. Ornstein, *Psychology of Consciousness.*

8. Johnston and Bauman, *Science and Religion.*

10. PRIMAL CONNECTION WITH THE SENSE OF TOUCH

1. Cohen, *Reconnecting,* 61.

12. PRIMAL CONNECTION WITH THE SENSE OF SMELL

1. Pandya, *Above the Forest.*

2. Endicott, *Batek Negrito Religion.*

3. Ibid.

4. Delon-Martin, et al., "Perfumers' expertise induces structural reorganization in olafactory brain regions."

5. Bushdid et al., "Humans Can Discriminate."

6. National Association for Holistic Aromatherapy.

13. PRIMAL CONNECTION WITH THE WORLD OF NATURE

1. Wheelwrite and Schmidt, *Long Shore.*

2. Woody Allen quoted in David W. Orr, "Quote of the Day: David Orr on 'Biophobia'," www.treehugger.com/natural-sciences/quote-of-the-day-david -orr-on-biophobia.html.

3. Kellert and Wilson, *Biophilia Hypothesis,* 42.

4. "Forest Bathing," Healthy Parks Healthy People Central, www.hphpcentral .com/article/forest-bathing.

5. Hess and Frolich, "Seven States Running Out of Water," www.usatoday.com/ story/money/business/2014/06/01/states-running-out-of-water/9506821/.

6. Statistics from the U.S. Geological Survey and the U.S. Environmental Protection Agency at http://water.usgs.gov/edu/earthhowmuch.html; http:// water.usgs.gov/edu/earthwherewater.html; http://pubs.usgs.gov/fs/fs2-00/;

and https://www.epa.gov/ground-water-and-drinking-water.

7. www.unwater.org/water-cooperation-2013/water-cooperation/facts-and
-figures/en/.

8. Goldenberg, "Why Global Water Shortages Pose Threat of Terror and
War," www.theguardian.com/environment/2014/feb/09/global-water
-shortages-threat-terror-war.

14. GOING DEEPER INTO PRIMAL RITES OF PASSAGE
IN NATURE

1. Metzner, *Unfolding Self,* 136.

15. PRIMAL MIND OF THE COSMIC CLOWNS

1. Kalweit, *Shamans, Healers, and Medicine Men,* 222.

2. Elgin, *Voluntary Simplicity.*

3. Fields, and Taylor, Weyler, Ingrasci, *Chop Wood, Carry Water.*

Bibliography

Bushdid, C., M. O. Magnasco, L. B. Vosshall, and A. Keller. "Humans Can Discriminate More than 1 Trillion Olfactory Stimuli." *Science* 343, no. 6177 (2014): 1370–72.

Cassirer, Ernst. *An Essay on Man: An Introduction to a Philosophy of Human Culture.* New Haven, Conn.: Yale University Press, 1994.

Cohen, Michael J. *Reconnecting With Nature: Finding Wellness through Restoring Your Bond with the Earth.* Corvalis, Ore.: Ecopress, 1997.

Delon-Martin, Chantal, Jane Plailly, Pierre Fonlupt, Alexandra Veyrac, and Jean-Pierre Royet. "Perfumers' expertise induces structural reorganization in olfactory brain regions." *NeuroImage* 68 (2012): 55–62.

Elgin, Duane. *Voluntary Simplicity: Toward a Way of Life That Is Outwardly Simple, Inwardly Rich.* New York: William Morrow, 1993.

Endicott, Kirk Michael. *Batek Negrito Religion: The World-View and Rituals of a Hunting and Gathering People of Peninsular Malaysia.* Oxford: Oxford University Press, 1979.

Endredy, James. *Earthwalks for Body and Spirit: Exercises to Restore Our Sacred Bond with the Earth.* Rochester, Vt.: Bear and Company, 2002.

———. *Ecoshamanism: Sacred Practices of Unity, Power and Earth Healing.* Woodbury, Minn.: Llewellyn Publications, 2005.

———. *The Flying Witches of Veracruz: A Shaman's True Story of Indigenous Witchcraft, Devil's Weed, and Trance Healing in Aztec Brujeria.* Woodbury, Minn.: Llewellyn Publications, 2011.

———. *Lightning in My Blood: A Journey into Shamanic Healing and the Supernatural.* Woodbury, Minn.: Llewellyn Publications, 2011.

———. *Shamanism for Beginners: Walking with the World's Healers of Earth and Sky*. Woodbury, Minn.: Llewellyn Publications, 2009.

———. *Teachings of the Peyote Shamans: The Five Points of Attention*. Rochester, Vt.: Park Street Press, 2015.

Fields, Rick, with Peggy Taylor, Rex Weyler, and Rick Ingrasci. *Chop Wood, Carry Water*. Los Angeles: Jeremy P. Tarcher, 1984.

Fonseca, Felicia. "Another Survivor of Sweat Lodge Retreat Speaks." AZCentral .com, October 21,2009, www.azcentral.com/news/articles/2009/10/21/200 91021sweatlodgedeaths21-ON.html.

Foster, Steven. *The Book of the Vision Quest: Personal Transformation in the Wilderness*. New York: Fireside, 1992.

Fredrickson, George M. *The Black Image in the White Mind: The Debate on African-American Character and Destiny*. ACLS Humanities E-Book, 2008.

Gerber, Richard. *Vibrational Medicine: The #1 Handbook of Subtle-Energy Therapies*. Rochester, Vt.: Bear and Company, 2001.

Goldenberg, Suzanne. "Why Global Water Shortages Pose Threat of Terror and War." The Guardian, February 8, 2014. www.theguardian.com/ environment/2014/feb/09/global-water-shortages-threat-terror-war.

Goodwin, Christopher. "At the Temple of James Arthur Ray." US News, July 8, 2011, www.theguardian.com/world/2011/jul/08/james-arthur -ray-sweat-lodge-arizona.

Green, Elmer, and Alyce Green. *Beyond Biofeedback*. Santa Barbara, Calif.: Knoll Publishing, 1989.

Hess, Alexander, E.M. and Thomas C. Frolich. "Seven States Running Out of Water." USA Today, June 1, 2014. www.usatoday.com/story/money/ business/2014/06/01/states-running-out-of-water/9506821/.

Highwater, Jamake. *The Primal Mind: Vision and Reality in Indian America*. New York: Meridian, 1982.

Hunt, Valerie. "Electronic Evidence of Auras, Chakras in UCLA Study." *Brain/ Mind Bulletin* 3, no. 9 (1978): 1–2.

Johnston, Lucas F., and Whitney Bauman, eds. *Science and Religion: One Planet, Many Possibilities*. New York: Routledge, 2014.

Jung, Carl G. *Psychological Reflections: A New Anthology of His Writings, 1905–1961*. Princeton, N.J.: Princeton University Press, 1953.

Kalweit, Holger. *Shamans, Healers, and Medicine Men*. Boston: Shambhala Publications, 1992.

Kellert, Stephen R., and Edward O. Wilson, eds. *The Biophilia Hypothesis.* Washington, D.C.: Island Press, 1993.

Linden, Wolfgang. *Autogenic Training: A Clinical Guide.* New York: The Guilford Press, 1990.

Luthe, Wolfgang. *Autogenic Therapy.* New York: Grune and Stratton, 1969.

Maslow, Abraham. *Religions, Values, and Peak-Experiences.* New York: Viking Compass, 1970.

Metzner, Ralph. *The Unfolding Self: Varieties of Transformative Experience.* Novato, Calif.: Origin Press, 1998.

Motoyama, Hiroshi, with Rande Brown. *Science and the Evolution of Consciousness: Chakra, Ki, and Psi.* Brookline, Mass.: Autumn Press, 1978.

National Association for Holistic Aromatherapy, www.naha.org/ explore-aromatherapy/about-aromatherapy/what-is-aromatherapy.

Ornstein, Robert E. *The Psychology of Consciousness.* San Francisco: Freeman, 1972.

Pandya, Vishvajit. *Above the Forest: A Study of Andamanese Ethnoamenology, Cosmology, and the Power of Ritual.* Chicago: University of Chicago Press, 1987.

Schultz, Johannes. *Das Autogene Training (konzentrative Selbstentspannung): Versuch einer klinisch-praktischen Darstellung.* Stuttgart, Germany: Geerg-Thieme Verlag, 1953. (In English: *Autogenic Training (Concentrative Self-Relaxation): Attempt at a Practical Clinical Presentation*).

Schultz, Johannes, and Wolfgang Luthe. *Autogenic Training: A Psychophysiological Approach in Psychotherapy.* New York: Grune and Statton, 1959.

Wheelwrite, Jane Hollister, and Lynda Wheelwrite Schmidt. *The Long Shore: A Psychological Experience of the Wilderness.* San Francisco: Sierra Club, 1991.

INDEX

BOOKS OF RELATED INTEREST

Teachings of the Peyote Shamans
The Five Points of Attention
by James Endredy

Earthwalks for Body and Spirit
Exercises to Restore Our Sacred Bond with the Earth
by James Endredy

The Journey of Tunuri and the Blue Deer
A Huichol Indian Story
by James Endredy
Illustrated by María Hernández de la Cruz and
Casimiro de la Cruz López

Plant Spirit Healing
A Guide to Working with Plant Consciousness
by Pam Montgomery

Plant Intelligence and the Imaginal Realm
Beyond the Doors of Perception into the Dreaming of Earth
by Stephen Harrod Buhner

Speaking with Nature
Awakening to the Deep Wisdom of the Earth
by Sandra Ingerman and Llyn Roberts

Plant Spirit Shamanism
Traditional Techniques for Healing the Soul
by Ross Heaven and Howard G. Charing

Becoming Nature
Learning the Language of Wild Animals and Plants
by Tamarack Song

INNER TRADITIONS • BEAR & COMPANY
P.O. Box 388
Rochester, VT 05767
1-800-246-8648
www.InnerTraditions.com

Or contact your local bookseller